# *The* Surprising Lives *of* Small-Town Doctors

• • •

**EDITED BY**

Dr. Paul Dhillon

 University of Regina Press

© 2016 Paul Dhillon

Printed and bound in Canada at Friesens.

Cover design: Duncan Campbell, University of Regina Press
Text design: John van der Woude Designs
Copy editor: Kirsten Craven
Proofreader: Katie Doke Sawatzky
Cover art: cover illustrations from the Noun Project: "Bear" by Loren Klein; "Stethoscope" by André Luis Gollo; "Sea Plane," public domain.

**Library and Archives Canada Cataloguing in Publication**

The surprising lives of small-town doctors / edited by Paul Dhillon.

Issued in print and electronic formats.
ISBN 978-0-88977-431-5 (paperback).—ISBN 978-0-88977-433-9 (html).—ISBN 978-0-88977-432-2 (pdf)

1. Physicians—Canada—Biography. 2. Physicians—Canada—Anecdotes. 3. Medicine, Rural—Canada—Anecdotes. 4. Rural health services—Canada—Anecdotes. 5. Canada—Rural conditions—Anecdotes. I. Dhillon, Paul 1981-, editor

R464.A1S87 2016   610.92'271   C2016-900160-1   C2016-900161-X

We acknowledge the support of the Canada Council for the Arts for our publishing program. We acknowledge the financial support of the Government of Canada. / Nous reconnaissons l'appui financier du gouvernement du Canada. This publication was made possible through Creative Saskatchewan's Creative Industries Production Grant Program.

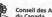
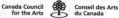

*To my Sarah*

# Contents

# Foreword

It is estimated that nearly 60 per cent of humankind will live in an area defined as urban by the year 2030. Not unsurprisingly, there has been a growing focus on the relationship between urbanization and health; our cities are busier, more auto-dependent, and more isolating than ever, which has driven up rates of chronic disease, mental health concerns, and societal upheaval. As economic and cultural drivers, cities attract enormous amounts of attention from governments to ensure that their contribution to nation-states continues uninterrupted.

Yet for countries like Canada, it is impossible for us to forget the swathes of population that live in remote and rural areas. From the vast frontiers of the Arctic and the North to the lush farmland of southern Ontario and the Prairies, Canadians by and large are defined as much by the hardy men and women in Prince Rupert and Cape Breton as they are by the frenetic pace of Toronto and Calgary. History, economics, and policy continue to sculpt the flows by which Canadians migrate, work, live, and play in our vast and diverse country, and these factors in turn influence their health and the nature of the health care they receive.

As a third-year medical student, I drove through northern Ontario to a rural rotation in family medicine and public health in Kenora, Ontario—a beautiful town where Winnipeg was the city, and where you could follow up your suspect flu cases just by shopping in the local Safeway. Rural living provided me with a different perspective on Canadian culture, history, and potential, and also on the essence of human nature. I imagine the stories in this book will do the same for you.

We are fortunate to live in a nation that, for those of us who call it home, affords us the freedom to choose from any number of tapestries on which our lives can unfold—from Arctic tundra to untouched coastlines, from boundless prairies to concrete jungles. The stories in this book celebrate not only our national identity but the national spirit that drives us ever forward, believing that in diversity lies our strength.

*—Dr. Lawrence Loh*
Associate Medical Officer of Health, Peel Public Health
Adjunct Professor, Clinical Public Health, University of Toronto
Director of Programs, The 53rd Week Ltd.

# Message from the Society of
# Rural Physicians of Canada

*A need to tell and hear stories is essential to the species* Homo
sapiens—*second in necessity apparently after nourishment
and before love and shelter. Millions survive without love
or home, almost none in silence; the opposite of silence leads
quickly to narrative, and the sound of story is the dominant
sound of our lives.*

—Reynolds Price, *A Palpable God*

Rural Canada is a breeding ground for stories. Rural medicine
is a fertile breeding ground for stories. When rural doctors and
patients get together, stories abound. When rural doctors get
together, the telling of stories becomes epidemic.

Patients use stories to illustrate their problems. An old trap-
per once told me, "I can still write my name in the snow when I
pee, but it's awfully close to my toes!"

Doctors use stories to help patients understand their diagnosis, treatment, and recovery. Inuit relate easily when told, "If
your son stops barking like a seal, his croup is getting better."

Doctors tell stories to other doctors to share adventures and
experiences. The Society of Rural Physicians of Canada (SRPC)
is the national voice of Canadian rural physicians. Founded
in 1992, the SRPC's mission is to provide leadership for rural
physicians and to promote sustainable conditions and equitable
health care for rural communities.

On behalf of its members and the Canadian public, the SRPC performs a wide variety of functions, one of which is fostering communication among rural physicians and other groups with an interest in rural health care.

Stories are the best way that I know of to communicate, and the hallways and lecture halls at rural conferences are alive with the sound of stories. We are always amazed at how well we can relate to other rural docs, whether Australian, South African, Kiwi, Pacific Islander, or many others. It is shared experiences and shared stories that make this happen.

I trust the stories in this book will contribute to the great practice of rural medicine and the even greater practice of storytelling.

—*Dr. Braam de Klerk, CM, MB, ChB*
Past President
Society of Rural Physicians of Canada

# Preface

For a writer, where does the physical book emotionally begin? In the case of this book, I remember the moment exactly.

It was a chilly but clear-blue-sky day in rural Saskatchewan. A phone call from the nurse had awoken me from my Saturday morning slumber and I trundled over the short drive to the hospital to see the patient who needed some care.

"It's really nothing," I overheard the sprightly ninety-two-year-old state emphatically as I was ushered into the examination room. "I don't see why you had to call back the doctor."

After introductions were exchanged, and sleep was wiped from my eyes, the story leading to the patient's arrival at the emergency department became clear. She was simply chasing away some stray cats from the milk she was putting outside for her cats and had slipped and fallen on her wooden steps. The resulting fall had not broken anything but had shorn a large area of tissue-paper skin off of her shin. As I was crouched down on the floor, carefully examining the large defect, I began some peripheral chatter about her living conditions and social circumstances. Surely she was not living out in a small wooden home in the middle of the prairies on her own at her age?

She continued her story as I patched and quilted my way around the wound, trying to repair the damage. She had been a war bride, had a life full of harsh winters punctuated with mosquito-ridden summers, had experienced immigrating to a new land, with all its pain and suffering and loss, and now had children scattered across Canada.

While doing my mending work, I realized in that moment that, as alone and isolated as a new rural physician can be, it is a gift to be able to share moments in the lives of Canadians, both recent arrivals and the long-established, that are shaping this great nation. Canada is a vast country, and as rural physicians, we are blessed with the challenges that this environment provides, in that we are given an opportunity to provide care for those that are the stitches and thread that bind together the patches of humanity that together make up Canada. In that moment I realized we are not the same without each other, and that without each other we cease to exist as a nation from coast to coast to coast.

That moment—when my patient shared her stories with me—is the place where this book emotionally began. And as I wrote out on her preventative medicine prescription, "stop chasing stray cats," I wondered if elsewhere there were physicians that felt the same way I did.

As it turns out, there are. There are physicians across the country silently sitting and listening to their patients' stories, empathizing with their pain, and then smiling at the successes of their quiet daily work. Unnoted beyond their communities, they continue silently. It was only after searching hard that I was able to find and pluck these individuals away from their work and to convince them to write openly—to share their secret fears and their individual moments of clarity and victory over the scourge of disease and the misfortune of injury. It took the guts of a year to find them, representatives from every province and territory of Canada. In some cases it was more happenstance than hard work that allowed this book to become the collection of experiences that it has become—such as a chance discussion with an American in the United Kingdom who happened to be married to a rural Quebec physician.

Now, almost three years after treating my elderly patient's shin, we have this wonderful tapestry of stories. Forty physicians in Canada, both old and new, have provided a pivotal piece of the ongoing narrative of what it means to be a rural physician in Canada.

Ultimately, however, the question must be asked—but why? Why is it important to share these stories? Are they of any value?

That question begins in the mind of the physician-writer and is answered by your thoughts today. Personally, I believe there is an intrinsic and therapeutic benefit to the physician as a human being to be able to express and share their thoughts with the interested public, which allows for both internal and, much needed, external reflection. Physicians are sometimes seen as being above the remit of normal emotions and life; should we not cry every single time we deliver bad news? In reality, though, we are human and suffer from pain like our patients. We have doubts and fears. We don't know everything. And we are tasked with some very difficult decisions.

Hopefully, through this book we are able to not only share those feelings and emotions with others in the healing professions but also with our most gifted assets, our patients. This book would not have been possible without the trust our patients place in our hands each and every day we go to work. Thank you for sharing your moments, your pain, and your stories with us; together, we are richer for the experience.

This project also would not have come to fruition without the thoughtful and respectably harsh comments provided by Dr. Tommy Gerschman. His comments are a reminder that behind the stories told by each physician lays a network of friends and family without whom these stories would never be told.

Lastly, names, identifying details, and places may have been fictionalized and/or changed in order to protect the privacy and rights of individuals throughout the book. In lieu of any royalty payments, the editor and the authors have agreed that all such proceeds shall go to *Médecins Sans Frontières*/Doctors Without Borders.

—*Dr. Paul Dhillon*

# Dr. Aedes Scheer

*Aedes Scheer was raised on a farm in southern Alberta and decided to become a veterinarian rather than a doctor after watching* Star Trek *and seeing the character Dr. Leonard McCoy treat multiple species. She became an animal health technologist, obtained a B.Sc., then tacked on a professional teaching certificate. She taught high school math and science for a few years and during this time she went to the Yukon Territory for a six-week vacation. Twenty-five years later, she still calls the Yukon home. While living in Dawson City, she provided veterinary assistance to the community, as there was no local vet; worked as a mosquito biologist (earning the nickname "Aedes"); served on city council; volunteered for the ambulance service; and started a humane society. She decided at age forty-two to go to medical school and began working as a GP in Dawson City in January 2013.*

## Friends and Neighbours

After several years of living and working in Dawson City in the Yukon, I decided to return to school to become a doctor. My accommodating husband and I did the long-distance thing for six years and, as I intended, returned to Dawson City. Prior to this new career, I had held numerous roles in the community. I was part of the town's fabric and possibly even a member of the heralded "Colourful Five Percent."

Although it was highly discouraged throughout my medical training, I maintained friendships with a large portion of my small community throughout med school and residency. As students, we were warned about the perils of getting too familiar with our patients. Sure, I understand that; I have heard it all before. Medicine is not my first profession. I was not a twenty-something med student—I could have given birth to many in my class—but I tend to view these sorts of things as guidelines rather than rules. I continue to see friends and neighbours in the clinic. I think this gives me an advantage when assessing patients. I know their "normal" because I see it displayed in the lineup at the post office and grocery store. I know sizeable chunks of their histories because I have heard these informally while helping put in a garden with a neighbour or sitting on the bench coaching their kids or standing next to them at a funeral. In my experience, people in small communities are accustomed to occupying multiple roles and while the occasional person wants to discuss a rash or some malady in a public setting, they clue in when I say, "How about you make an appointment on Monday?"

I had volunteered with our ambulance service for several years prior to starting medical school. I saw many excellent doctors and nurses arrive in the community but then leave when the lack of anonymity became too much of a burden, or it was too difficult to find a spouse in a diminishing pool of people not yet seen in the clinic. The flipside was that when doctors and nurses stayed completely apart from the townspeople, they missed out on knowing the people they treated. On more than one occasion I recall bringing a local in to the nursing station and reporting that something was not right with the patient. I couldn't quite put a finger on it, but they were not the person I knew in the day to day. This was often dismissed as interesting but lacking evidence. And, inevitably, the person was medevacked out for something that just needed time to evolve. It began to dawn on me that because I was comfortable living in the small town, plus my spouse was comfortable living there too, maybe I could learn how to be a doctor, and then possibly become a doctor who did not leave.

Small towns being small towns, Dawson's population is somewhat incestuous. We have a saying, "fall together, spring apart"; relationships often form for the cold months but break up once the light and warmth returns and the greener pastures of transient summer workers appear around town. Consequently, Dawson City is tolerant of nontraditional families and a wide spectrum of lifestyles. I first learned about this when I was providing veterinary services on a house-call basis and was asked to euthanize the aging family pet. I would show up to a diverse house full of grieving people all associated with the doggy I was about to put to sleep. By the time I packed up my bag and expressed my last sympathies, I had some additional insight to all the combinations of couples and kids who had been a part of the dog's life. The years of house calls and comforting pet owners have provided valuable background information, as well as ample bedside-manner training, for me in my current role as a GP.

However, just when you think you have the upper hand, do not get too smug. Medicine is utterly humbling and will remind you how little you really know. Even about yourself.

One day, while newly back in town as a doctor working a twenty-four-hour, on-call shift every second day (a "1-in-2 on-call"), the ambulance pulled up with a good friend of mine on-car. He was weak and short of breath and found to be in a narrow complex tachycardia. Bob is a big guy in his mid-forties with a past history of hypertension, smoking, and heart disease with a stubborn paroxysmal cardiac arrhythmia. His vital signs were still holding strong and we tried a couple of doses of adenosine.

This did not change anything. We were about to try metoprolol, as had been done in the past for him, when his vital signs tanked. Now we needed electricity. I tried to explain to him what was going to happen next as the nurse got things ready for an electrocardioversion, but I was not sure he could hear me. To my surprise, he reached out and grabbed my hand and said, "Aedes, I know you so well I can hear in your voice that you are scared and that is scaring me." Yep. He nailed it. I was scared for him and I couldn't hide it, even though he was failing quickly. Tears ran down my cheeks and I could not shut them off. He started to cry too. And then, voila! His heart rate settled, his blood pressure resumed a textbook reading, and he sat up. We were wiping away the tears and grinning sheepishly when the nurse walked in. She sort of squinted and clucked under her breath but announced our patient had spontaneously cardioverted.

I had assumed that I had the advantage; I know my patients and therefore I can give them better care. The thing is, they know me too. Apparently, I don't have a "poker face" when it comes to my friends. I could try to fake a brave front, but that does not seem honest to me. I have decided not to bury what I am feeling. It is a better approach, and I am finding that if I am up front with my emotional state and my patients, I am not caught off guard as I was with Bob. Like fraternizing with our patients, in med school we were counselled against being emotionally transparent with our patients. But then, my patients are neighbours and friends, the very group of people my medical school said we were not supposed to see as patients. So maybe two negatives make a positive? I don't purport to be anything but human and am therefore subject to the weaknesses and strengths of that species. I am finding there may be little difference between these and that an apparent weakness can become a strength.

# Dr. Sarah Giles

*Sarah Giles is a geographical error—she was born and raised in Toronto—but she likes to say she hides it well! After completing an undergraduate degree and medical school at Dalhousie in Halifax, she moved to Thunder Bay for residency in family medicine at McMaster University. She has spent the past eight years working as a locum in northwestern Ontario, the Northwest Territories, and Western Australia. In 2013, she completed her diploma in tropical medicine and hygiene and almost immediately put those skills to work in 2014 working for* Médecins Sans Frontières/Doctors Without Borders *in Myanmar, South Sudan, and Pakistan. In 2015 she successfully challenged the emergency medicine exam. She writes a column for the Medical Post called* YoungMD *and a blog for Canadian Healthcare Network (www.canadianhealthcarenetwork.ca) called* Point of Care: where life meets medicine.

## In the Middle of the Night

"Doctor Giles! *Doctor* Giles! *Doctor Giles!*"

I tried to figure out who was calling my name. Why was someone screaming my name? Where were they? Where the hell was I? It was all too much to process from the depths of my sleep.

Then it suddenly all clicked. I was in a remote Arctic community doing a community visit. It was the middle of the night. Somewhere in the bed and breakfast I was staying at, someone was frantically screaming my name. I don't think I'd ever been called with that sort of urgency before. Flinging my door open, I found a man dressed in winter gear at the bottom of the stairs. "We need you at the health centre right now!" he implored. I grabbed my glasses and hurriedly started to throw on clothes. Remembering that there was a resident doing the community visit with me, I started to yell his name. "Stephan! Stephan! Get up!" Which room was he in? Screw it, it didn't matter, the entire building must be awake. "*Stephan!*" He emerged from his room, his outrageous curls flopping everywhere. "Throw on some clothes! There's some sort of emergency. Let's go!"

In the Suburban, we got the briefing: a woman had fallen down a flight of stairs and the nurses said she wasn't doing well. I was eighteen months into my career in rural and remote family medicine and I was scared. Luckily, though, I had somehow scored a great resident (who felt much more like a colleague than my student). Shit. Shit. Shit. It was going to be us or nobody. I took a deep breath and tried to stay calm. Could I fake the confidence and skills required to save this woman? I wasn't sure.

When we walked into the room, I knew things were bad. The woman was collared and struggling to breathe. ABCs. ABCs. "Start bagging her," I said before even taking off my jacket. Her heart rate and blood pressure were good, but she looked terrible. She was bleeding from the head. "Put in an oral airway." Shit, she didn't spit out the airway—she had lost her gag reflex. "Sarah," one of the nurses said, "check her pupils—they are sluggish." She was right. By this point, I was swearing out loud.

"Have you called for a medevac? Okay, I'll do it," I said as I watched the resident perform the secondary survey.

"We will need to intubate this patient. What drugs do we have?" I had just done the Difficult Airways Course in Boston and was ready to use all the fancy drugs, but none of them were in the tiny health centre.

"Ativan and midazolam" was the reply to my question. Neither of those drugs was on my algorithm for intubation.

As I spoke to the doctor at the referral centre, requesting a medevac, he told me there was actually one on its way to a neighbouring community and that they could reroute it. The critical care nurse and paramedic would have all the drugs we needed. I sighed in relief.

"Sarah, the patient's blood pressure is getting really high. And have you noticed that one side of her chest is much higher than the other? I think she has a pneumothorax. I can't hear breath sounds on one side." I thanked my lucky stars for having an amazing resident. We quickly needle decompressed the patient's chest—the "whoosh" of air was just like they said it was going to be in the textbooks—and her vitals stabilized.

Within ten minutes of calling for a medevac in a remote Arctic community, I had the flight team by my side with drugs drawn up. "My angels with wings!" I cried as they had entered the building. That sort of response time is unheard of in remote regions of Canada. Perhaps things would be okay after all?

As I sized up the patient for intubation, I knew it was going to be tricky. As a staff person, I hadn't actually intubated anyone and now I faced a collared patient! Using the bougie and scrounging up all residual courage, I got the tube on the first try. A wave of relief flooded my body. I realized that I had sweat through my clothes.

"Sarah, the patient's BP is going up again and I can't find the catheter we used for the needle decompression. I think it fell out." *Shit.*

"Repeat the needle decompression and prepare for a chest tube," I told the resident, chastising myself for having failed to better secure the catheter.

I called the regional trauma centre to let them know about the patient I was sending them. "It doesn't look good."

With the chest tube, endotracheal tube, Foley catheter, and multiple IVs in place, men from the community carried the patient, on the stretcher piled high with a ventilator and tubing, out to the plane. I breathed a sigh of selfish relief—we had gotten the patient out of the community and she was alive, but I knew that she likely didn't have long to live. She would get a CT scan and then the doctors in the big centre would deal with whatever needed to be done. I had done my part.

But I wasn't actually done. A few hours later, I received a call from the doctor at the referral centre. The patient's injuries were not compatible with life. A decision had been made to send the patient back to her home community so she could be extubated and die surrounded by her family. I begrudgingly accepted the patient—I was not sure what sort of care she would need and I was concerned that the tiny health centre would not be able to meet her palliative needs. Although I understood the desire for the patient to come home, I also desperately wanted to sleep. I wanted the problem to go away. I was exhausted and had used all my skills to keep her alive, and now I was being asked to do the opposite.

As the medevac team touched down in the community once again, people began to flood into the health centre. There were more people than I could count. Once again, they lovingly carried their friend and relative over the snow and into the health centre. I addressed the family, who then asked me to address the crowd.

"Mrs. Smith has suffered a severe brain injury. Right now, she is only alive because the machines are breathing for her and supporting her vital organs. The family believes that she should be allowed to die a natural death. I will give you all time to say your goodbyes to her before we remove the machines. Once the machines are removed, she may continue to live, but I do not think it will be for very long. Please, take your time." I felt help-less. I had tried to keep this woman alive, we all had, but I had failed. And now there was an entire community looking at me. I wanted to run.

I removed myself to the corner of the patient's room and watched as what seemed like the entire community filed past her bed. After everyone had said their goodbyes, a family member asked everyone to gather into the room. "I would like to say a prayer," he announced. His prayer asked for God to take care of his family member and the usual sentiments one hears in this situation. As an atheist, I listened quietly and respect-fully but in a rather detached manner. That is, until I heard the following: "And, God, thank you for Dr. Giles. Thank you for bringing her to us and for allowing her to give our family member a chance at survival. We are grateful for her effort and her compassion."

I was stunned. The family and the community weren't angry with me. They didn't think I was incompetent. They were actually thankful for my presence. I wondered how such grace was even possible.

As I tried to discreetly brush away my tears, the people filed out of the room. Without needing to speak to one another, I quietly stopped the pump for the IV pressors. With that, the patient's heart rate and blood pressure quickly rushed to zero. We extubated her and removed all of the tubes that had invaded her body. She was returned to her natural state.

I opened the door to the room and informed the family that she had died the moment we turned off the machines. As they filed past me, the men shook my hand. My body shook with attempts to control my sobs. They were, however, no longer sobs of shame and failure but of relief and thanks.

That day, I realized that perhaps there is more to medicine than saving lives, especially in remote environments where phys-icians usually aren't present. If we happen to be there and give a patient the very best shot at survival possible, maybe that's the best we can do. The people in this community appreciated the harsh reality of life in remote regions, but I was just beginning to understand it.

# Dr. AnneMarie Pegg

*AnneMarie Pegg took the "life experience" route to medical school—entering after working as a nurse in both the big city and rural Northwest Territories for several years. Her lack of ability to decide on a single specialty meant that rural medicine was a natural fit. She has been working in various communities in the Northwest Territories since finishing residency in 2006. For the last several years, she has divided her time between rural locums and international work with* Médecins Sans Frontières/Doctors Without Borders. *She finds that the flexibility, adaptability, and ingenuity that serves her as a rural physician has also been invaluable in her work in some of the most difficult places in the world.*

## Whack!

A few memorable letters and other correspondence I have written during the years I have practised in the North have stuck with me. There is something I find fascinating and often entertaining about the interface between the truly unique situations I often find myself in and the twenty-first-century medical care offered in our referral centres. There is a paragraph in my most favourite consult letter that goes something like this:

*The patient states he was examined by the nurse, who also performed a cardiogram, and then quickly left to get the doctor. He recounts that on arrival, the doctor looked at the cardiogram, spoke briefly to the nurse, and then "turned around and punched me really hard in the chest," after which he felt significantly better.*

That is pretty much how it went. It had been the last day of one of my fly-in clinics to the isolated communities in the region, a visit that had already been extended by one day due to bad weather, which had prevented the landing of the plane that was supposed to take me back home. I had been watching the sky all morning, willing the fog to dissipate in order for me to be home for the weekend.

My patient, let's call him Bob, was in his mid-thirties. He had previously been in excellent health. He had apparently woken up and gone to work as per his usual routine. However, partway through his workday he was overcome with a sudden sensation of weakness, dizziness, and shortness of breath. A colleague had brought him to the health centre. He was quickly assessed by the nurse. His blood pressure was barely recordable, he was pale and diaphoretic, and his ECG was something one rarely sees: a complete twelve-lead cardiogram of ventricular tachycardia, which meant the heart muscle was contracting in a very dangerous rhythm.

I recall instructing the nurse to ensure he was in the major treatment room so we could cardiovert his heart with an electric shock immediately. And I clearly recall her response: "We don't have a defibrillator here."

There have been a few moments in my career when I have completely stopped in my tracks with the same feeling as I experienced that day: *What. The. $%£$. Am. I. Going. To. Do. Now?*

I also have somewhat of a strategy to deal with this situation. I call it my "Put on your big girl panties and figure something out" approach to difficult situations. Over the years, it has served me generally well. However, I had less experience applying that strategy in my first year of practice than I do now.

Back to Bob. A small part of my brain recalled learning about sudden disruptions in cardiac electrical activity causing death, and about precordial thumps (strikes to the sternum), possibly in one of those history-of-medicine lectures, when we are taught about the barbaric and non-evidence-based things our predecessors did. I remember the voice of one of my clinical instructors as well: if you're going to do it, don't warn the patient, hit them as hard as you can, and you only get one chance.

I—calmly, I like to think—disconnected a few of the ECG leads that were still attached to Bob's chest. I mentally land-marked the area I would aim for.

I turned my back, ostensibly to recheck something in his chart, but in reality it was to take a deep breath and convince myself this was a reasonable course of action and that I wasn't about to do something that would land me in court so soon after my career had begun.

And then I did it.

I punched him really hard in the chest.

When my fist made contact, I could hear someone in the room yell. It could have been Bob. It could have been the nurse. And let's face it—it quite possibly could have been me.

And then I took my stethoscope to listen to his chest. I could barely manoeuvre it. I was probably as diaphoretic as the patient. *What if it hadn't worked? What is the success rate of a precordial thump, anyway? What are the common complications? Has anyone done any research on this? If I end up in court, is this going to be upheld as a "reasonable act by a group of my peers"? Does this nurse think I'm a lunatic? The patient most certainly does. Maybe I should have tried something else first?*

And then I heard it—*lub-dub, lub-dub, lub-dub*. Regular. Not muffled. We reconnected his ECG leads.

Normal sinus rhythm: ninety-two beats per minute. Significantly slower than my own heart rate at the time.

I remember smiling at Bob and telling him his heart rhythm seemed to have returned to normal. I apologized for hitting him. I explained the physiology behind the gesture. I expressed my own gratitude for the fact it had worked.

He thanked me for the explanation and said he felt better and would like to return home. I explained it was a bit soon and that he would still be medevacked to a hospital for investigations as to why this had occurred in the first place. I discussed ongoing care instructions with the nurse. We made arrangements for the transfer. I called ahead to the referral centre to explain the case. The senior resident I spoke to sounded both fascinated and horrified. It was clear, however, that the patient likely wouldn't have survived a transfer, which would have taken an hour or more, in his previous state.

The fog had cleared as well. Planes to transfer Bob to definitive care, as well as me to my house, were both able to land that morning.

And I am happy to report that the health centre is now equipped with a defibrillator.

# Dr. Courtney Howard

*Courtney Howard hails from the mist and moss of North Vancouver but grew up dreaming of the sparkling North where her parents met and fell in love. After medical training and work throughout Canada, as well as work with* Médecins Sans Frontières/Doctors Without Borders, *she moved to Yellowknife where she now works as an ER physician and lives with her pediatrician husband and two daughters. The heart-wrenching bedsides of acute medicine have given her an appetite for prevention, and she has realized that climate change is a threat held in common by northern Aboriginal populations and mal-nourished African children, as well as one likely to affect the quality of life of current Canadian kids. She therefore works with the Canadian Association of Physicians for the Environment (CAPE) to use the uniting power of our shared desire for good health to rally doctors and others towards a sustainable world with a human-friendly climate.*

## Arctic Data Streams: Graphing Land and Love

We were standing around talking about water in the staff room at Inuvik General Hospital when I realized I'd been picturing the ocean emptying into the river. Flushed with "Thank goodness I didn't say that out loud!" med school–shaming angst, I looked again at the wall-mounted world map, studded with colourful pins denoting the far-flung hometowns of Inuvik's medical learners, and tried to figure out how I'd mentally ended up with a subconscious assumption that the Beaufort Sea flowed south into the McKenzie River—instead of the other way around. I blame gravity. If you flicked water at a map hanging on a wall, it would flow south. How embarrassing—an unexamined, completely backwards thought.

A few minutes later, the locum obstetrician, the one whose dictations still make me laugh when I come across them in old charts in the Yellowknife ER ("I told her no screwing or ski-dooing for two weeks!"), breezed through our conversation on her way to the OR and exclaimed, "Oh! I thought it ran south. I wonder why. Ha!"

I smiled, wondering how many Canadians operate with gravity-based geography.

I think of this seven years later as I squeeze past people at the entrance to the meeting hall in Yellowknife and scan for a free seat amidst all the puffs of down jackets. I slot myself into one of the few chairs left and introduce myself to the older Dene man on my right. His hand is warm and dry.

"You're not with the coal people are you?" he asks, raising an eyebrow.

"No. I'm a local doc."

"A what?"

"An emergency medicine doctor. From Yellowknife."

He eyes me. "Good."

We sit in silence. I spot some city counsellors, some MLAs, the chief officer of public health, a friend who works in media. The head family doc in town rushes in looking harried. Everyone is here because they're worried about our water quality following the spill of a coal tailings pond into the Athabasca River, upstream. Having grown up in the anonymity of Vancouver, I'm still unused to being able to pick so many people out of a crowd.

"This spill." My neighbour turns towards me. "This spill is no good. We'll see more like these. I live on the land. I've lived on the land since I was a boy. Last spring, a lake that had been there my whole life poured into the river."

"Really?"

"Yep. The land that was separating the lake from the river just melted away and the river drank the lake. Global warming. People don't know these things. People who don't trap, who don't travel on the land, don't know these things."

These stories always hit me somewhere close to my solar plexus. "That must have been upsetting."

"Yes. Things are different."

*Solastalgia.* The word glides through my mind. It's a word I've learned recently, described in studies into the mental health effects of the changing climate on the Inuit. It means feeling homesick while you're still at home. *Solastalgia.*

He looks sad. "Everything is different. So I've come to hear what they have to say."

"It looks as though a lot of people feel the same way." The room has become so crowded they slide back the partition to expand the space.

Five people sit at the head table. Two government scientists, two Aboriginal leaders, and a representative from the coal company. The rep goes first. Young, pleasant. They sent him alone. He describes how they knew that the berm of the coal tailings pond had been breached the evening that it happened, that they had been unable to contain the spill, and that the tailings had travelled the length of a small stream and emptied into the Athabasca. They had done "everything possible" to monitor it, but, of course, it was freeze-up, which made for difficult conditions.

His company is very concerned. They are a "sustainable coal mining company." Two chairs away from me, a hoot of laughter.

Our local Rhodes Scholar covers her mouth quickly, as though surprised the sound had escaped.

Next, the water scientists. Very well respected. They've been following the spill and the turbidity is approaching baseline levels. No problem for the drinking water of the North. The chief medical officer is called upon to speak—he is reassuring. We all nod at the graphs. Raising my daughters as I am on the shores of Great Slave Lake, I am pleased.

Finally, the man who has been sitting in a pool of quiet at the head table rises to speak. He is the leader of the Aboriginal group just downstream from the spill in Alberta. He thanks everyone for their information, nods at the coal company rep, says he respects him as a human for coming. The poor young man from the coal company looks miserable for the first time.

Despite the fact that the leader's eyes are cast down and he seems to breathe in fatigue, something about him makes us lean in. A palpable sense of responsibility, gracefully shouldered. My own breath slows, is almost held, as he speaks.

"They've never been faced with a serious situation like this before. They felt like their man-made dykes wouldn't fail. The provincial government doesn't know what they're doing. The federal government doesn't know what they're doing. This tailings pond was constructed fifteen years ago. So it was a new tailings pond that breached. We have thousands of older ponds." He continues, describing how his people still fish on the river, still live traditionally as much as they can. Meanwhile, the accumulating development projects in his area are changing the landscape so much as to make it almost unrecognizable.

He looks up. "We are going to be environmental refugees because of environmental catastrophe occurring on our land."

By now we have tears in our eyes. And one by one, other leaders stand to speak. They are from upstream and downstream, their home communities connecting the dots of my medical life in the North, bringing images from that life to mind.

Aklavik—sprawled in the coatroom of the health centre, trying to reduce a Husky's partly frozen, prolapsed uterus as the head nurse strokes her fur. Fort Simpson—on the phone with their nurse, standing at another map, this one in the Yellowknife ER, running a code over the phone, measuring the distance the medevac has to travel against the number of ampules of epinephrine the nurse has left to administer. Fort Good Hope, Fort MacPherson. Stories of the land, of time spent outside on sparkly snow, of fish and traplines, of hopes for their children's future on their land. As the leaders speak, my mind's eye wanders up and down the river system. Fort Providence—a Chipewyan-speaking Elder is brought in with constipation and gets tired of waiting for the translator. He suddenly bursts out, "No shit!" and raps the table next to his chair, causing the loudest explosion of inappropriate laughter of my career.

Finally, an Elder with a long braid stands. He says, "This is the problem. These people have a low spiritual IQ. So when they pollute the water, that's not a problem to them."

We have all heard words like this before, but it is this man's tone that grips me. He is not angry or braying or accusatory. It takes me a second to place the sound, like a tune heard out of context. Finally, I realize it is the same tone that is used by medical mentors as they try to explain the cultural differences relevant to practising in a given context. When we say things like, "Remember, in the Far North they may say 'yes' by opening their eyes wide. Be ready for that. Do what you can to adjust," we use the same helpful tone as this Elder. He is earnestly trying to explain a cultural gap, to create a space for understanding.

I have never been in a room where I am part of the cultural group that is being explained.

He continues, "We who know the land, we have a responsibility to ensure that they look at the land more spiritually."

He presents no graphs.

Spirituality. Turbidity. *Solastalgia.*

Stories. I have recently realized that although doctors think that we make decisions based on evidence, much more often we change our practice based on the story relayed along with the evidence—based on the efficacy of an epinephrine drip in a code ran over the phone and the success of polyethylene glycol in a single, extremely constipated, Chipewyan Elder. We respect numbers, but, for better or for worse, we follow stories.

Such a big map. On such a vast map, the few lines mean a lot. Up here, in a land of few roads, those lines are our waterways. Those lines connect us, those lines make a community of our little pockets. Up here, with fewer people, we have time to hear people, to be named. We know who is in the room, we know what resources we have, we know better when we may need to stand up. In a way, as we are named, we are called.

As I shuffle out, nodding at my neighbours and winding my scarf back around my neck, I spot a lapel pin, frequently seen in these parts, that says, "Love the land."

It has been here the whole time.

I step into a crystalline night, considering the potential of love as an ally to my graphs. And I wonder whether I will soon realize that other parts of the world have been flowing backwards on my mental map.

**NORTHWEST TERRITORIES**

# Dr. Adil Shamji

*Adil Shamji is a Toronto-based family physician with a particular interest in the care of vulnerable and underserved populations. Since completing his residency in 2013, he has practised in settings ranging from barren landscapes in the Canadian High Arctic to fast-paced emergency departments in urban trauma centres. He is a faculty member at the University of Toronto, and has a number of interests including medical education, advocacy, and aviation.*

## Fear and Fantasy above the Arctic Circle

It had been two hellish days. Two days of sharing my personal space with strangers, of constantly sitting down then standing up, of frantically running from one terminal to another as I caught a series of flights that took me progressively farther and farther north. Walking through airports, my massive Canada Goose parka had elicited stares and sneers from passers-by, who each assumed I was an entitled city boy living from the coffers of affluent parents. They were right to some degree—I *am* from Toronto—but they did not know that my parka was about to serve a function far more important than making a fashion statement on Yonge Street.

I was headed to the Arctic.

Just six months earlier, I had completed my family medicine training at the University of Toronto. Before that, I had received my undergraduate medical degree from Toronto as well. I was prepared for anything. I had seen the weird, wild, and wonderful things that a University of Toronto education provided, and I was trained to become an instant expert in anything else by intensely examining the literature when the situation demanded. These were lies I was telling myself, of course, but I willed myself to believe them so I could rise above the confusing turmoil of emotions I felt below.

Fear. Excitement. Self-doubt. Determination.

Nothing could stop me and, yet, anything could.

In fact, something already had. Mere months previous, on my first day ever as a licensed physician, I had been the only emergency doctor at a hospital in a remote Aboriginal community. The day had gone disastrously, with a young man barely older than myself dying from septic shock and a woman suffering a cardiac arrest at an even more remote community that was attended only by nurses. The nurses had called me for help and I had guided the resuscitation over the phone, but to no avail. For days after those deaths, I had dreaded coming to work, fearing that similar events might repeat themselves. With the tincture of time, those wounds had slowly healed and I had come to realize that I could not and would not have done anything differently. Yet the same doubts always returned whenever I travelled to a new location for work.

Four months after that disastrous day, I was on the final flight of my journey to Inuvik, Northwest Territories. Inuvik is a small town located two degrees above the Arctic Circle and is home to the most northern hospital in Canada. I knew very little of actual substance about Inuvik, and instead had been drawn there by romantic notions of mystery, adventure, and danger. My mother's alarm when I initially proposed the idea had only strengthened my resolve to carry through with it, and during moments of doubt I had been buoyed by thoughts of polar bears, Arctic explorers, and the chance to see first-hand the fabled Northwest Passage that connects the Atlantic and Pacific oceans. At the same time, I looked forward to being spared the tedium of downtown Toronto walk-in clinics and the chance to practise the full scope of family medicine—including obstetrics, in-patient medicine, and emergency medicine—in a community that genuinely needed physicians.

As my flight descended into Inuvik, so, too, did the sun. I was landing in Inuvik on December 6, the final day of sunlight before the town endured thirty-one days without sunrise. In the airport, a man in bright coveralls who noticed me standing alone grabbed my bags and offered to drive me wherever I needed to go. My instructions had been to call a cab and arrange my own transportation to the hospital, so my urban instincts screamed at me to call for help, or grab my bags back, or, at the very least, politely decline his offer. However, a nearby RCMP officer seemed unperturbed as he watched the scene unfold and something told me to take a chance. It turned out the man was a local hydro worker who was concerned that I looked lonely, confused, and out of place in the terminal. I had heard of southern hospitality, but no one had mentioned anything about the Far North.

Upon arrival, the work in Inuvik arrived quickly and consistently. Within hours of being received at the hospital, my pager went off. A man had been stabbed in the chest in one of the remote communities. All the other doctors were occupied. Would I go there by air ambulance and place a chest tube? I couldn't, I politely declined. I hadn't even received my hospital privileges yet.

Shortly thereafter, a young woman stopped me in the hallway.

"I'm the public health officer here," she told me. "What do you know about botulism? We just had a case here a few weeks ago and I want to make sure you're prepared."

Botulism!? I thought back to what I had learned. I remembered it was a life-threatening bacterial infection that released paralysis-inducing toxins. These toxins were commercially used in the form of Botox to remove wrinkles, combat excessive sweating, and relieve migraines. Clinical botulism was not a problem that I had ever heard of in Ontario and, surely, none of my friends had either. A diagnosis like that would have made the evening news throughout the province.

She must have seen the quizzical look on my face because she offered an explanation: "People home-can their own fermented seal blubber here, and if there are any mistakes in the canning process it can allow botulism to proliferate."

Ahhh. How did U of T forget to teach me this?

My time in Inuvik was divided between family medicine, emergency medicine, in-patient medicine, and obstetrics. Each offered its own unique challenges and rewards. Family medicine above the Arctic Circle consisted of many of the same clinical problems my Toronto patients had but with a uniquely northern flavour. For example, all children had to undergo a vaccination series to protect them against the usual infectious diseases—measles, mumps, rubella, etc. However, children in Inuvik also received a vaccine to protect them against tuberculosis. This immunization—the infamous BCG vaccine—was a ninety-year-old treatment instituted to protect against TB in vulnerable populations. I had never known it to be administered in Canada and, yet, here it was. To support this vaccination program, public health did a splendid job of keeping meticulous records of their patients' immunization status. In this and other ways, I was surprised to learn that medical practice in the Northwest Territories was in many ways more efficient and streamlined than in Toronto. Of course, this was not always the case. As a trainee at U of T, I had the good fortune of being able to offer my patients almost any diagnostic test or treatment. In Inuvik, ubiquitous tests that I had been trained to rely on such as musculoskeletal ultrasound or MRI were nowhere to be found in the entire territory. I was forced to return to William Osler's methods of taking a detailed history and performing a thorough physical exam.

Emergency medicine in Inuvik proved to be particularly rewarding, in part because I had many opportunities to vindicate myself of those earlier deaths from my first day in practice. Each shift in the emergency department was a harrowing mix of sick patients in parallel with multiple telephone calls to offer support to the excellent nurses who operated medical stations alone in our remote communities. On some shifts, hours could go by without a patient to be seen. Other shifts transformed our small emergency department into a formidable ICU. On one occasion, two patients arrived almost simultaneously with life-threatening gastrointestinal hemorrhages that called for emergent transfusion. Our hospital, stocked with eight units of blood, had barely enough to replace the blood loss in one of them. Years of preparation had taught me how and when to transfuse but had not prepared me to choose who should live or who should die. The question had been posed in our ethical training, to be sure, but the reality of overabundance had never forced me to make, or even observe, how such decisions would be made. In the end, both patients depleted our entire stock of blood and were transported by Learjet to Alberta. And somewhere in between all that, I performed a lumbar puncture on a seven-day-old baby.

The adventure I sought came in droves. I drove by ice road to a community of only 150 people and, while returning, lost control into a snowbank nearly two metres deep. Stranded on a patch of road many kilometres from any habitation, I was able to call the RCMP for rescue using a satellite phone. Weeks later, the RCMP would help me again while on Banks Island, in the most northern community of the Northwest Territories. Noting my disappointment at having not yet seen a polar bear, I accompanied them on a snowmobile patrol of the island to see if any could be found. We searched for hours in temperatures that dropped well below -40°C, but the bears still eluded us. The patrol culminated in a mad dash across the frozen Arctic Ocean to ensure I would not be late for home visits that I had yet to perform in the community.

Although I returned from the Arctic without ever having seen a polar bear in the wild, I came back with experiences that were far more rewarding. I saw the northern lights. I endured thirty-one days of darkness. I crossed the Northwest Passage to reach Banks Island. As I did these things, I discovered new cultures and encountered amazing people from all walks of life. Some had lived their entire lives in the North, and others had been drawn by the prospect of work, adventure, or the chance to make a difference. Although the medicine was unique in its practice and challenges, the motivation that compelled us to see our patients was the same in the Arctic as it was in Ontario, or anywhere else in Canada. Our patients were sick, and we wanted to be there to cure sometimes, relieve often, and comfort always.

# Dr. Kyle Sue

*Kyle Sue has been a full-practice, general practitioner locum and clinical assistant professor in Nunavut since completing his rural family medicine residency at Memorial University in 2014. A quarter of his residency training was done in Nunavut, with the other three-quarters in Newfoundland. He is active in ultrasound teaching at Memorial University as a Canadian Emergency Ultrasound Society (CEUS) independent practitioner and master instructor.*

## Do Not Feed the Polar Bears

*Ulaakut!* (Good morning!)

So what is it like being one of approximately fifteen physicians at any given time covering thirty-seven thousand people over a two-million-square-kilometre land mass? There is no way to do it justice with words, so while I will share a few stories with you, I urge you to go there to discover its wonders for yourself.

A quarter of my family medicine residency training was in Nunavut, as part of the brand new NunaFam program. While there have been countless residents up here before me, nobody prior had the privilege of spending six months here during residency. I have a great love for rural medicine, particularly in the Arctic. Although as a medical student I had spent a month at the Inuvik Regional Hospital, the only hospital in Canada above the Arctic Circle, it still did not prepare me for some of the surprises and challenges of working in the Arctic as a physician.

### When Evidence-Based Medicine Doesn't Exist

We were having a bit of a rough week as the sole in-hospital physicians. Post-surgical patients, newborns, children, the acutely psychotic, the suicidal, heart failures, pneumonias, tuberculosis—you name it, we looked after it.

This week, all of the hospital beds were full, from the obstetrics beds to the ward beds to the emergency room beds. Hospital administrators were rupturing an aneurysm, metaphorically of course, trying to get us to discharge or transfer whomever we could. "Transfer the sick kids! They're much easier to sell!" No, administrators were not referring to child slavery. "Sell," in this case, refers to how bad you could make a patient's condition sound to the accepting physician for a patient transfer to the city.

On the hospitalist service, we are also responsible for taking calls from nurses concerning any patients walking into a remote community nursing station where there are no physicians. In fact, out of the twenty-five communities in Nunavut, only three have any full-time physicians. All of the other communities rely heavily on phone consultations with physicians from hundreds to almost two thousand kilometres away.

One afternoon during this rough week, I received a call from a remote nursing station about two brothers who were attacked by a polar bear. Apparently, the two brothers were out on the ice floe edge hunting narwhal. When they were asleep in their tent, a hungry polar bear tore it open and gnashed his teeth into one brother's scalp. While the bear was dragging the man out of the tent by his scalp, he somehow had the presence of mind to grab a Swiss Army knife from his pocket, which he repeatedly jabbed in a backwards motion into the bear's head. The bear let go of him and decided to go for the other brother instead. The bear swung his paw into the other brother's back, completely shattering a shoulder blade. Meanwhile, "Mister Open Head" managed to scramble to grab their gun to shoot the bear dead. Problem solved, right? Nope. They were 250 kilometres from the nearest remote nursing station, which was another 1,200 kilometres from the nearest hospital. After a few hours on their snowmobile, they reached the nursing station, where the nurses called our hospitalist service in a panic.

The nurses cleaned the wounds, bandaged them up, and got them on a medevac plane. The plane finally landed back in Iqaluit by late afternoon, and the men were brought immediately to the emergency department. Upon arrival, Mister Open Head asked the emergency physician if he could go outside to stretch his legs. The two men were certainly much calmer than we expected! Mister Open Head was stitched up with over a hundred stitches, his tetanus immunization was updated, and he was given some Advil. The CT scan of his head did not show any internal bleeding and no major fractures. Mister Broken-and-Bloody Back apparently only needed "a sling for comfort," according to the consultant orthopedic surgeon in Ottawa I had phoned, despite the shoulder blade being in multiple pieces on imaging.

So now I'm left with a decision on what to do. I certainly could not admit them to the in-patient unit—they were both too stable, and we were full anyways. I wondered if there were any evidence-based studies for treatment of polar bear attacks. If there is evidence for treating "seal finger," there must be some evidence for what antibiotic to use for polar bear bites and scratches, right? Nope, I could not find anything online on the subject. I called public health, which also did not know what antibiotic to use, but they suggested giving rabies prophylaxis, as there was a case of rabies in a polar bear twenty years ago. I decided to treat it like a simple cat or dog bite, and gave the brothers oral amoxicillin-clavulanate…to go. I told them to come back in the morning after a couple days to get checked, to make sure nothing was infected. I questioned my decision not to give them intravenous antibiotics, but fortunately no infection ever developed. They also did not require anything stronger than Advil for the pain! For once, I even offered to give them something, but they both said that the Advil was working fine. It just goes to show how tough the Inuit are! Neither of them felt particularly traumatized by the incident—instead, they now had an impressive story they could tell for the rest of their lives of how they fought off and beat a polar bear!

This incident made me think about how I would defend myself if a polar bear ever came after me. I sometimes work in Qikiqtarjuaq (Qik), a community of 250 people on Broughton Island, just north of the Arctic Circle. In Qik, I have been advised by the nurses not to wander around town without a firearm, as polar bears regularly roam the town. I have never held a firearm in my hands, so that was not an option for me. Fortunately, years of Coca-Cola commercials have taught me that if I offer the bears a bottle of Coke, I will earn their trust and cuddly friendship. We'll see how that goes…

### NunaFamous

When I first moved north, I had no idea what to expect. Nobody told me I should pack two thirty-kilogram suitcases full of food and alcohol to bring up there. Food is expensive and variety is poor, though, fortunately, there is an authentic shawarma shop run by Lebanese owners, who deliver to me while I am on call. Alcohol is not easily purchasable. All hamlets in Nunavut are dry, and it is a criminal offence to possess alcohol, except for in Iqaluit, which is a "damp" town. A damp town is a town where you can buy alcohol at restaurants and bars, which have quantity restrictions, or buy alcohol for special occasions if you have applied for and received a permit.

I was confused once when I was unable to find vanilla extract on the shelves of the local supermarkets to feed my baking habit. Turns out it is a controlled substance as it is 70 per cent alcohol—the same as mouthwash. I substituted ginger ale for white wine in my cooking. I once brought back beer from Greenland. These unique circumstances led me to create a guide to outline everything I wish I had known prior to coming up north, and everything I would want to know when first settling in. Since that hilariously inaccurate guide was produced, it has apparently been passed on from person to person and has made its way through town. Word has it that the RCMP now offer it to their new constables. In 2014, when I went back for my second stint in Nunavut, strangers I had never met referred to me as "the Kyle," as in "the Kyle who wrote the guide."

### "Sorry, Doc, There's No More Antibiotics in Town…"

When I am not physically in Nunavut, I am on the regional on-call schedule for the Kivalliq region, which is essentially the mainland part of Nunavut. This entails being the consultant physician—from a distance—for 450,000 square kilometres, covering most communities other than Rankin Inlet, which has a full-time physician living there. This can entail dealing with anything from a septic pre-term labour (early labour due to a full-body infection) to a simple urinary tract infection.

During one shift, I received a call from a nursing station regarding a four-month-old infant with a "simple" urinary tract infection detected by a urine dipstick. The baby had stable vital signs, a very mild fever, and still had good oral intake. She was just a little more irritable than usual. Unfortunately, this infant had serious allergic reactions (anaphylaxis) to any penicillin-like antibiotic. What did we have at the nursing station? Only penicillin-like antibiotics. They had run out of any other usual oral antibiotic used for urinary tract infections, except for an adult double-strength pill of Septra, which obviously would be too high a dose for an infant. They did have intravenous gentamicin, but there was no way to monitor the drug level as the nursing station had no laboratory capabilities. If the drug level is too high, it could lead to kidney failure and permanent deafness. It was also a long weekend, so the nearest pharmacy, a two-hour flight away, was closed. I had four options: 1) use an antibiotic that is typically ineffective in urinary tract infections; 2) give nothing, and wait out the long weekend, crossing my fingers that the infant would not worsen in the meantime; 3) give intravenous gentamicin for a very mild urinary tract infection, probably malpractice; 4) fly the infant out on a medevac plane at a cost of over $20,000 to taxpayers.

I ended up choosing option two. I figured if the child got a lot worse in the next couple days, I could then justify the cost of flying the child out (assuming good weather and the availability of a flight team). On Tuesday morning, I quickly faxed a prescription to the pharmacy in Rankin Inlet, and it was flown on a scheduled flight to the remote community by late afternoon. Fortunately, the child did fine. I only pulled out a few chunks of my hair that weekend from fear and frustration.

This reminds me of the time when a community ran out of the anticonvulsant that a patient with a seizure disorder required...but that is a story for another time.

So, have I convinced you to sign on the dotted line to visit or work in the North? I certainly love it!

*Qujanamiik!* (Thank you, goodbye!)

# Dr. Charlie O'Connell

*Charlie O'Connell worked at the Distant Early Warning (DEW) Line Base from 1955 to 1956. The exact address was Site 30, Fox Base, Hall Beach, Melville Peninsula, Northwest Territories, now a part of Nunavut. It was at sixty-nine degrees latitude and eighty degrees longitude, code: APO864; Charlie Fox Charlie 500. His medical practice extended from Cambridge Bay in the west to Rowley Island near the shore of Baffin Island, a distance of about a thousand kilometres. His work included many distant flights to other bases and Inuit igloo areas, including the Fox General Hospital: three beds and two mattresses.*

## Igloo House Call

"Marconi" Ron rushed to Fox Hospital with a telegram:

> *Inuit baby born yesterday. Baby okay. Afterbirth not come. You come please Doc.*
> > *Ches Russell, Hudson's Bay, Repulse.*

"Ron, please ask the airstrip if the plane is ready for Repulse," I asked.

"Okay, Doc. Right away."

From the DC-3 cockpit the pilot shouted in his Scottish accent, "Come aboard, Doc!"

I boarded with my limited medical kit and we taxied down the icy runway. A relatively smooth flight with a bumpy landing through icy air and air pockets did not bother Gallagher's perfect landing at Repulse. I was greeted as we disembarked the plane.

"Thanks for coming, Doc. I'm Ches Russell, Hudson's Bay," said a pleasant weather-beaten man who greeted us. "An Inuit woman needs your help. We'll drive the snowmobile as far as we can and then meet the Inuit dog team."

An Inuk in parka and mukluks waited with his team and *komatik* (sled).

"This is Ikpik, Doc. His wife Salika is your patient," Ches said.

"The doctor will remove your wife's afterbirth," he followed in Inuktitut.

Ikpik stood on the komatik runners, cracked the whip, and the huskies were off. I gripped the sled as lead dogs jumped a one-metre crevasse. The next dogs in the tandem fell into the icy hole but were rescued by the lead dogs pulling their harnesses.

We crashed over shore ice near Ikpik's village home—we had arrived at my first igloo house call!

Inside, caribou skins made the floor look cozy; more skins covered the raised sleeping area. Flame from a whale oil pan gave heat and light.

Salika cuddled her newborn and kissed her husband a welcome home.

I opened my medical bag for sterile gloves, administered Salika an analgesic, and completed a manual removal of her retained placenta.

Blood clots gushed out with the placenta. My hands, from inside and outside, massaged and hardened the uterus. No more bleeding.

Ikpik threw the placenta to the huskies and made tea and bannock treats. He calmly chewed frozen seal meat.

I enjoyed Inuit hospitality, but not the cuisine.

I received a letter the next week, translated from Inuktitut:

*Thank you Medicine Man. Wife and baby good. Ikpik.*

I treasured that letter, along with mitts, mukluks, and memories of the Canadian Arctic. DEW Liners risked their lives during the Cold War but also learned to admire and love our stoic northern Canadian neighbours, the Inuit.

# Dr. Madeleine Cole

*Madeleine Cole is a family doctor who lives and works in Iqaluit, Nunavut. Despite growing up in downtown Toronto, she is the anomaly who has found professional and personal happiness in a small northern community. She has a longstanding commitment to sexual health and reproductive rights and remains passionate about improving the health of Inuit. She has a full-scope clinical practice at Qikiqtani General Hospital and is director of medical education for the region. The hospital has a partnership with both Memorial University and the University of Ottawa and many family medicine trainees come to Iqaluit for elective rotations in Nunavut. Health ethics is another professional interest of Madeleine's and she has led the creation of a hospital ethics committee in Iqaluit. If she is not at the hospital, she is likely playing on the tundra with her partner, Kirt, and her kids, Noah, Jayko, and Naja Jane.*

## A Room with a View

Pausing outside the sliding glass doors of the emergency department, hands on her hips and leaning slightly forward, she tucked her chin, closed her eyes, drew four, long, slow breaths in through her nose, and then entered. Clad in a long, shapeless raincoat but with a telltale waddle, she approached the clerk's desk and waited in the pool of water that had accumulated around her soggy sneakers.

Nothing in Peter's face betrayed the fact that when a woman in labour arrives at a hospital without Caesarean section backup, doctors get nervous. As they walked to the examining room together, perhaps my mentor, a smart, compassionate, and cautious physician, hoped to find that she was in false labour. Or maybe she would be early enough on as to allow us the four-hour window that, weather permitting, would allow for a medical evacuation to a more resourced setting. No such luck. As an enthusiastic medical student on an elective on this remote northern island, I had yet to appreciate the headaches and worry involved in arranging medevacs.

It was a week before Mary's due date, or thereabouts. A plane ticket to the big city had been given to her two weeks before during a clinic visit where we had explained, again, that the town's hospital was not equipped to manage deliveries and that the risks to the baby and herself were substantial if problems arose during the birth.

It would not be the first or the last time I would experience resistance to the advice that we health-care professionals felt would be "in the mother's best interests": leave your community and await your labour in a city that has more services. Who can blame Mary for having opted to give birth in a room whose immense window faces east across the ocean chop to the snow-capped mountains? As beautiful as it was, I am wise enough to understand that it is not the view that makes most women want to give birth close to home.

This was Mary's second baby and according to her cervical changes, if her progress remained smooth, we would be hearing the wails of a new life in less than three hours.

The reality of an imminent birth moved us from angst to action: we would expect a healthy birth but prepare for a scarier scenario. We reacquainted ourselves with the resuscitation equipment: checked the oxygen flow and the intubation equipment and made sure the drugs were not out of date. Beside the warmer, the protocols for managing flat babies were stickytaped to the wall. "Flat" is the odd term we use to describe floppy newborns that are having trouble breathing or, worse yet, whose hearts are not ticking along at a hundred or more beats per minute.

As luck would have it, Michelle, a doctor who used to work in the North, was back for a locum after having completed training to do Caesarean sections. With Peter and Michelle assisted by my helping hands, and the extra nurse we called in, if we absolutely had to, we could pull off a Caesarean section.

As is the case in many small rural hospitals, the operating room had been shut down since the days of the jack-of-all-trades outpost doctor. When it comes to moving sick patients, our contemporary transportation woes are nothing compared to the days before phone lines and the lonely airstrips that litter northern communities. The small-town doctor had to be able to do C-sections; she also had to yank out inflamed appendices and rotten teeth, release incarcerated hernias and testicular torsions, and face other such eventualities that required the knife.

Unaware of our contingency plans, Mary changed into a blue hospital gown and called her husband to tell him the day had come. In time with the rhythm of her own internal sea, she slowly walked the length of the corridor, stopping to crouch as her contractions built up painfully and then washed away.

In less than two hours, I was guiding the soft, warm body of a beautiful, wrinkled baby girl into the outside world. Outside the rain had stopped and as the late afternoon sun dropped below the clouds, it created a brilliant streak across the water running from the glowing mountains to our beautiful island hamlet. When her intact placenta followed the babe a few minutes later, a collective sigh of relief dissipated into the happy air.

Mary gave a tired smile and a look that seemed to suggest she had known all along that everything was going to turn out just fine.

• • •

Today, my home is in a land of great beauty and vast geography that currently has the highest birth rate in the country. Across three vast time zones are scattered twenty-six small communities; three of which have birthing programs and one of which has an operating room. Pregnancy and birthing care remains one of the greatest challenges and joys of rural and remote medicine. We become a part of the intimate story of new life, and at times also share in great sadness. We try hard to keep families together, to reflect on the real risks in any given situation, to be cautious and educated, and to share decision making with women. We strive for happy, healthy outcomes. Recalling my formative experience twenty years ago on the Inside Passage brings peace and perspective to my daily challenges.

**NEWFOUNDLAND AND LABRADOR**

# Dr. Kyle Sue

*Kyle Sue received his M.D. from the University of Alberta in 2012 and his B.Sc. from Simon Fraser University in 2008. He grew up in Delta, British Columbia, and is a proud Seaquam Secondary grad. He is known for his generous, caring personality, his amusing anecdotes, his passion for travel, and his nine lives. He is concurrently completing a master's degree in health management and three years of fellowship training in developmental disabilities, pain medicine, and palliative medicine in Ontario, Nova Scotia, New York, Alberta, and British Columbia.*

## The Gambo Gamble

Newfoundland is the definition of friendly. Although I am a CFA (Come from Away)—in other words, a "Mainlander"—Newfoundlanders have been the most welcoming people I have ever met.

"I've lived in eight provinces and territories—I can drive in anything," I reassured myself as I turned the key to start my car. It was a snowy night with blustering, eighty-kilometre winds in St. John's. I had signed up for a continuing education course in "Gandahar" for the next couple of days. Gandahar isn't the town's real name—it's just what medical residents affectionately call Gander, in reference to the large Canadian Forces base there that we compare illogically to the one in Kandahar, Afghanistan. Gander is a small town in central Newfoundland, about 350 kilometres west of St. John's on the moose-filled Trans-Canada Highway. Gander was put on the international map when planes to New York were diverted to the Gander airport during the 9/11 attacks. News reports widely covered the generosity of families in Gander who housed, fed, and clothed complete strangers from those planes. The reason I decided to do the course in Gander was twofold: 1) they had available spots; 2) it was complimentary for employees of the health authority, which included medical residents. Rather than wait for a spot to open up in St. John's, I only had to go a few hours out of my way to get it done faster and for free. The hospital also agreed to pay for my accommodations while there, so why not?

Unfortunately, the weather decided to take a turn for the worse, which happens often out on the Rock. We laugh at stories of people reporting their cars missing only to find them exactly where they had parked them when the snow melts in the spring. The snow can be so heavy that the shape of your car will have completely disappeared from sight overnight, and the wind is so habitually strong that even one measuring 100 km/h does not keep people from leaving the house. In fact, 100 km/h winds are pretty typical.

A couple of hours into my drive, I had zero visibility with the blowing snow. The road was white; the sky was white; everything was white. I didn't care about looking out for moose like I normally did on such drives across the province—I just needed to know where the road was. Every couple of seconds a post with reflective markers would come into view to signal the edge of the road. It dawned on me that driving to Gander that evening wasn't such a good idea after all. It was probably this

"I can handle anything" mentality, along with Newfoundland's frequent inclement weather, that resulted in four out of thirty-three of my family medicine classmates destroying our vehicles in accidents that year on these treacherous roads. Whether it was moose, hydroplaning, snow, or sheer bad luck, far too many of us got into motor vehicle accidents that year. This is despite having all-wheel drive and winter tires. Soon four became five...

After about an hour and a half of zero visibility, all of a sudden I could see the road begin to curve left, but my car continued to head in the same forward direction despite what my arms and the steering wheel demanded of it. Stomping on the brakes in such weather is never a good idea, but what about the parking brake? Too late. There just wasn't time to think. In the blink of an eye, my car flew off the road and began to flip forward. I felt a strange calm as this was all déjà vu—I had flipped my car off a Yukon mountain in a similar manner a few years back while on a rural elective rotation as a medical student. Boom. Crunch. Splash. *Splash?* That was not a familiar sound. As I hung in my car upside down, suspended in mid-air by my seat belt, the car's cabin began filling with water from the rear. I pressed the red button on my belt buckle to undo my seat belt and dropped onto the inside of my car roof. The car was tilted in such a way that the rear was in water and the front remained dry. While I swung the car door open, I could see a man scrambling down the thick, snow-covered embankment. I could make out the shadows of his family behind him at the top as he asked me what he could do to help. In the next minute, I tossed him a suitcase, a backpack, insurance papers, eyeglasses, and my autographed Dan Mangan CDs that had been floating in the rear of my car. He grabbed my arm and helped me up the embankment. When I got to the top, I looked back to see that my car was floating upside down in a riverbank. This was the Gambo River. Although I no longer remember what the family looked like, I do recall that the father, mother, and two young boys were standing out in the blizzard, looking concerned as they made sure I was all right. It turns out the father was an off-duty paramedic who had taken his family to watch a movie in a neighbouring town that evening, despite the snow!

I don't know how, but I felt completely fine. *No injuries!* I thought to myself.

"Ya gots an 'uge black h'eye 'n some scratches on yer face," said the man in his central Newfoundland accent, "better get ya an h'ambulance." I actually would have had no idea how to call an ambulance or the police, as there is no 911 service in Newfoundland outside of St. John's and Corner Brook. I did not know what the local emergency service numbers were.

"Umm…the black eye and scratches are from yesterday. I had a fall at home…It's been a bad weekend."

Meanwhile, I looked around and noticed that a few other drivers had stopped at the side of the road and were wading through the snow towards us. Despite it being midnight, all four families kept me company in the blowing snow and we laughed at my misfortune that weekend while waiting for the RCMP to arrive. They all offered to drive me the remaining fifty kilometres to Gander, despite it being out of the way for all of them. It was one hundred kilometres out of the way for one family! I decided to wait for the RCMP to arrive before figuring out the next steps.

When the RCMP officer arrived, he offered to tag team with officers in neighbouring detachments to deliver me to my destination. I thanked the four families and wished them a safe journey as I hopped in the passenger seat of the RCMP pickup truck. The officer was originally from small-town Quebec, but he had been living in Gambo, Newfoundland, for the past five years. "Even the bad guys here are nice and friendly," he commented, "I'm staying here for good."

A few rides later, I arrived at the James Paton Memorial Hospital in Gander. I walked into the emergency department to ask for the keys to my pre-arranged apartment. Turns out, there was some clerical error and they didn't know I was coming. The triage nurse reassured me, "Don't you worry. I'll call the hotel for you. We'll have it billed to Central Health. If you need anything, don't hesitate to ask! You can have one of the hospital vehicles if you need to get around." The service made me feel like a guest at a five-star hotel, but, alas, it was just normal Newfoundland hospitality.

Before I walked away from the desk, the nurse glanced at my black eye and asked, "Are you sure you don't want to see a doctor before you go?" I laughed and shook my head. Now was not the time to tell the story of my weekend.

• • •

B'y, I tells ya—da' warmth o'Newfoundlanders do melt yer 'eart. (Translation: Boy, let me tell you—the warmth of Newfoundlanders will melt your heart.) Not only does it melt your heart, it also keeps you warm when you're standing outside in a blustering blizzard.

This warmth instilled in me a burning desire to stay in Newfoundland for good, much like that Quebecois RCMP officer. It doesn't matter if you're a CFA—you're still welcomed by strangers as if you were a good friend, neighbour, or family member. Perhaps the helpfulness of strangers is something prevalent in any rural location in Canada, but I'm convinced that Newfoundlanders are a unique brand of friendly that surpasses anything I have experienced elsewhere. Even in the isolation of that frozen snowbank, there was a heartfelt feeling of togetherness as my extended Newfoundland "family" passed the time with me, with laughter, joy, and plentiful conversation.

# Dr. Kelly Anderson

*Kelly Anderson completed a postgraduate degree in international project management and spent nearly a decade working in the non-governmental HIV/AIDS sector before seeking more training through medical school. She completed a fellowship in HIV medicine through the Ontario HIV Treatment Network and is now a family physician at St. Michael's Hospital, within the Department of Family and Community Medicine at the University of Toronto. Beyond her general and HIV primary care practices, she is a part-time emergency physician in Georgetown, Ontario. She spends every free minute enjoying time with her two little boys.*

## Invisible Resources

A darkening sky filled with falling snow, a fierce wind across my face, the whir of snowmobiles echoing in my ears, sounds muffled by my hat and hood. Crinkling snow pants. Warm hands in mittens, stuffed in pockets. Short fir trees masked by snowdrifts. Walking slowly up the road, pulling each boot up out of the snow, one at a time.

Stepping through the doorway, my wet boots track snow over the cardboard flooring. Many other pairs of boots line the entry, and voices filter through from the next room. Unzipping my coat, I turn to the living room and notice the hands of a small, elderly woman being held. Someone is telling her a story in a low-pitched tone. Scanning the dimly lit room reveals at least twenty others. The arctic cold does not penetrate this space; it is warm and inviting. Family portraits hang, crowding one another on the walls.

This is a home visit to a dying woman in a northern Inuit community in Labrador. It feels silly to play doctor in this moment. Despite the stethoscope around my neck that indicates a certain purpose, I am mostly just a witness, an outsider. With so many eyes on me, I find myself trying to say some reassuring things. They seem somehow miniscule compared to the care I see and feel in the room that will carry this woman through her final moments. I am in awe, having never seen so many people present for the death of a loved one.

I am left thinking how powerful such a gathering is: they will each take turns, holding her hands, telling her she is loved, telling her stories of her life and her family. Her friends tell me about what she was like as a child. Her children reflect on what a strong figure she is as a grandmother. I watch the visitors take care of her household: cooking, bringing food, cleaning, tending to the day-to-day necessities of the family. I feel privileged to watch this happen for the days on end that I visit. I feel like I am being educated about belonging, about having your entire personal history be firmly situated in one geographic place. About being thoroughly known and, in this case, appreciated by neighbours.

I have heard some remote northern Canadian places referred to as "low-resource." I understand this terminology from a material perspective. I have witnessed many financial and physical limitations in housing, water supply, and health-care provision. I don't wish to minimize the challenges faced by some northern communities because I don't have the experience to fully understand them. I know that the singular experience I witnessed is not a universal one, nor does everyone get to experience belonging to a community just because they are rural or remote.

But it strikes me there are other, sometimes-ignored resources in places deemed "low-resource"—ones we don't see readily as outsiders. This singular experience in the North, among many others, gave me the opportunity to feel strong community in a visceral way. Is connectedness to community an invisible resource? Does strength of community impact health outcomes? How can we celebrate and promote the more invisible, health-fostering strengths, the ones we don't measure within the norms of urban, Western medicine? Do these strengths go unrecognized, unappreciated?

At home in Toronto, weeks later, I stand in my apartment at night, watching a darkening sky full of falling snow. I see bright street lights and cars speeding by below me, a take-out sushi place flashes with neon lights. I'm separated from pedestrians below by thick glass windows and cement walls. In the background, my bright laptop screen blinks with incessant emails and social media demanding attention. It occurs to me that I don't know any of my neighbours beyond casual greetings. I could reach out a kilometre in every direction and not know anyone to a significant degree. Although there is deep connectedness in pockets of this city, and many striving to build more community, there can be a striking isolation despite our physical proximity to one another. Are we "low-resource" when it comes to connectedness and community?

I have been fortunate to train in and practise family medicine in the most urban places and some of the most remote. Having seen the benefits of strong community on health, I wonder if there may be a connectedness deficit filtering down into how we practise family medicine in big places. Am I the type of doctor who stops to really listen? Or am I impatient, overly busy, or too overscheduled to be in that place of receptivity? I could spend most of each appointment typing about the encounter into the computer health record. Some days I am too desensitized, exhausted, or detached to take the extra minutes to ask about a family member, listen to a story, or chat with a colleague about the day. How can we build more connection into the way we practise, and what differences could it make?

Although I learned the scientific tools of medicine in school and residency, it reminds me that I entered family medicine to answer a different question for myself: How do we build the most healthy and resilient communities? How can I be a part of that no matter where I am? My experiences in the North have, so far, given me the best glimpse of doing this. I can see that by educating myself within strong communities, and seeing how they can influence people positively, I have the opportunity to make connections stronger; to call on aspects of communities that can help individuals through health challenges. But it demands a higher level of openness, and a willingness to keep my eyes open to the potential invisible resources I have not necessarily been taught to see.

# Dr. Nicole Fancy

*Nicole Fancy is a Halifax, Nova Scotia, native, now living in Prince Edward Island. She is currently in family practice, in-patient care, and emergency medicine in the town of Montague. Completing her undergraduate studies at Mount Saint Vincent University in biology, chemistry, and religious studies, she then went on to medical school at Dalhousie University. After medical school, she completed her postgraduate family medicine residency in Prince Edward Island, and has since been happy to make it her home, together with her husband, Steven.*

## Interpretations of Opioids and Raccoons

September 24, 2012. Monday morning. Time to start another week. I remind myself that at least I'm not on call. The emergency room still gives me anxiety. I am late getting to the office because I had a complicated new admission over the weekend, and I just spilled coffee on myself in the parking lot. Grab a chart and get moving.

"I am originally from Halifax. Yes, I am old enough to be here. And, yes, I plan on staying," I say with a smile as I shake Mr. Gallant's hand.

As I met each new patient in my practice, they all had the same three questions before getting to their particular health concern, and those were my answers. After months of meeting new people, I began giving the answers before the questions were even asked, as I knew they were coming. Asking where a person is from and if they have "Island" connections was always the first question on their lists. Addressing their shock at how young I look tended to be the concern behind question number two. And the most important question, would their new doctor be just another to quickly come and go?

Montague is in eastern Prince Edward Island. The catchment includes various smaller, primarily fishing or farming, communities. The patients I have taken on have been without a steady family physician for about ten years, and they are scared I will come and go as many have before. This is an intimidating way to start a practice. Even if you do plan on staying, the constant reminder of the commitment is nerve-wracking. It also happens to be wildly fulfilling to directly address a need of so many people and to feel so appreciated.

Between making this major commitment and realizing how many of my new patients had suffered from a lack of consistent primary care over the last decade, it was clear that this new role would not be easy. The initial few months are challenging for new physicians: trying to apply all the medical knowledge from training to the highest possible standard while simultaneously working to gain the confidence of colleagues and building rapport with patients. There is the desire to be a good doctor and at the same time the wish to be liked by the community.

Perhaps the most challenging encounters are when these goals seem at odds with one another. What a patient may expect and want from you is not necessarily the best thing for them according to evidence-based medicine. Pain management is a common clinical scenario where this takes place. Sadly, rural communities are often plagued with addiction issues and limited resources to manage them. As the green new grad, how do you address the many patients you inherit who are on chronic prescription narcotics for unclear purposes, knowing how doctors are often blamed for creating the current state of prescription-drug abuse across the country? Luckily, like most challenging situations, the small victories can make the struggles feel worthwhile.

One of the local pharmacists called to tell me about a new patient, Mrs. Blue, whom I would be meeting later that day. He was so excited she had a doctor and hoped I would address her pain management. Mrs. Blue was a woman in her early sixties who he feared was chronically overdosing on acetaminophen and codeine. She had been taking eight Tylenol No. 3 pills a day since her last doctor left, getting the prescription refilled at walk-in clinics. In addition, she was supplementing with Tylenol No. 1 and regular Tylenol, and was often in requesting more for her pain. She had led a tough life, with a history of chronic depression and a strong family history of addiction.

She complained of pain everywhere. Her low back was worst. She complained of chronic nausea and no appetite. She had almost no facial expressions. Her eyes had a deep sadness, and she shied away from eye contact to conceal it.

With each patient, you manage the best you can. You try to manage them as individuals, with the best mixture of communication skills and medical knowledge you can muster. You can often only hope you have done a decent job. You ask screening questions, looking for any red flags before you reassure them, as you end up doing during most visits.

Most family doctors have multiple Mrs. Blues in their practice. There are many variations of her, but at first glance she is much the same. During one visit with Mrs. Blue I realized she had on a beautiful bracelet and nice blouse. She had a smile on her face. I reflected on the fact that she physically looked brighter than on that first day we had met. I complimented her but was somewhat surprised by her response.

"Oh, I'm glad you like it. I only get dressed up when I come here to see you," she said with a smile.

I wasn't sure how to interpret this: Should I be flattered that she felt seeing me was an important occasion? Sad that these fifteen minutes spent together were work for me but a highlight in her week? Or should I view her outfit as just strictly evidence of how little she was getting out and socializing?

The fact is, there is merit in each interpretation. I now know she enjoys our visits and values my opinion. I also know that she remains isolated and has a poor quality of life most days. I know my attempts to help her change this have been only minimally effective thus far.

After I had complimented her, she smiled right away. We then chatted about her family. I mentioned a seniors visitor program that might interest her. From there we talked about some enjoyable things she could do with them. We adjusted her pain medication and set a few goals and arranged to meet again in a few weeks.

This is one of the beauties of family medicine, and the beauty of making Prince Edward Island my home. There is plenty of time to work on these difficult cases. Like most people in our society, doctors typically like when things are quick and easy to fix. Unfortunately, complex problems rarely have simple solutions. Thankfully, the relationships we are able to build in family medicine can be of great help when tackling these challenges. And the small victories, like gaining some trust, can be an important step along the pathway to addressing the larger issues.

In addition to being important clinically, the interesting encounters we have with patients are paramount in making this profession so unique. As a family physician, you never know what you may hear when you walk into the next exam room. People trust you and tell you things that are not a part of usual conversation. Being a rural physician can colour these encounters even more.

The rural emergency room brings no shortage of interesting experiences. Treating animal bites is a relatively common clinical experience. Medical students can rhyme off the bacteria *Pasteurella multocida* as the bacteria to cover for when selecting an antibiotic to treat a cat bite. On one occasion, when an elderly man came into the department with his hands covered in bites, I figured another feline was to blame.

"It was a raccoon. He must not have recognized me," the elderly man explained matter-of-factly as I came into the room.

"Recognize you?" I wasn't sure where this encounter was headed.

The efficient side of me, which was acutely aware of the full waiting room, contemplated not probing any further and just getting directly to treating the bite and deciding whether or not this man was at risk for rabies. And if he was, what the heck was I supposed to do about it? But the comprehensive and perfectionist side thought perhaps he needed an MMSE (mini mental state examination) or a delirium workup if he thought he was communicating with raccoons. Just this simple scenario and remark had my brain scattering in different directions.

"Well, yes, I always feed him. He usually lets me pick him up. He purrs just like a cat, you know?" He said this with a laugh as he pretended to pat a cat in his arms. "I jus' got outta hospital today. Had knee surgery you see. Coming along good. Was in for almost three weeks, had a little set back. He just didn't recognize me, poor fella. I scared him. I shoulda figured."

I guess there is nothing inherently wrong with feeding wild animals. Interesting choice. Still, I got a nurse to call his family and confirm this was normal behaviour for him. First, I politely asked for his permission to do so, which gave him a good laugh. The family, who corroborated his story, and I both had a good chuckle, too, in the end.

I have yet to experience a dull day in my new position. With the truly unique and interesting scenarios, alongside the

conquered challenges, rural family medicine is a truly privileged position. While it can be both difficult and exhausting, I
feel grateful every day for the opportunity I have to call family
medicine my profession, and to call rural PEI my home.

**NOVA SCOTIA**

# Dr. Monika Dutt

*Monika Dutt is a public health physician and mother living in Cape Breton, Nova Scotia. She is the medical officer of health (MOH) for the Cape Breton District Health Authority and a family physician in Wagmatcook First Nation. She has lived in Cape Breton, with her four-year-old son, since July 2012. Previous work since finishing her public health and preventive medicine residency in 2008 has included being an MOH in northern Saskatchewan, a health policy analyst for a Member of Parliament, the chair of Canadian Doctors for Medicare, and taking on family medicine locums in many northern settings.*

## Toy Truck

I stand in front of the Cape Breton Regional Municipal Council, co-presenting a policy proposal that will support breastfeeding in the local area. To my right is the dais where the mayor and high-level civil servants sit. On the screen behind me is the slide I am speaking to. It lists the many reasons breastfeeding is good for health—and it is normally a simple task to review them. Good for mother, good for baby, good for the environment. Done.

But today my back is damp with sweat and I lose track of my place on the slide. It is difficult to stay focused as a two-year-old runs a toy truck over my head. Back to this scene in a moment.

I moved to Cape Breton to be the medical officer of health (MOH) in July 2012 with my son Kail, who was one at the time. I made the big decision to move here spontaneously, the way I often make significant life changes. After finishing my residency in community medicine, now public health and preventive medicine, I spent two years in northern Saskatchewan. I was based in La Ronge, a town of two thousand, and worked with First Nations and Métis communities throughout the North. After that I worked on health policy with a Member of Parliament. The beauty of public health is that you can "practise medicine" in many ways—MOH is a formal, typically specialty-requiring position, but public health happens, well, everywhere.

There had been no one full-time in the Cape Breton MOH position for many years. No competing for limited big-city jobs for me—it seems almost unfair that I have always wanted to work in places with hard-to-fill positions. It's like a secret pleasure—if all those other new grads realized how fun, interesting, and challenging it is to work in small communities, I'd have a lot harder time finding work.

Given the lack of a recent MOH, I felt both exhilarated and intimidated at being able to shape my job. There are, of course, programs, policies, legislation, and job requirements to follow. Yet, given that public health hinges so much on an understanding of the local community and striving to address health issues that can range from housing to poverty to the potential health impacts of fracking, the opportunities for personal approaches are endless.

There is also a satisfaction in knowing that anything I do, in and out of work time, to learn more about the place I have chosen as my new home will also help me as MOH. That includes attending a ceilidh filled with live fiddling in Judique, touring a replica mine at the Miners Museum in Glace Bay (with weathered ex-miners as guides), and eating dinner made with local food ingredients at Flavor restaurant in Sydney—all of these activities reveal information about factors that shape health such as culture, employment, and food.

Working in public health at the local level means being part of translating the day-to-day issues people deal with to policies that can benefit many; for example, if one woman feels uncomfortable breastfeeding in public, what can we all do to ensure women who are breastfeeding feel supported in any setting? To complement that work, I continue to practise family medicine and spend one day a week in a clinic in a local Mi'kmaq health centre. Maintaining a sense of how the individuals I see in the clinic connect to their community is essential grounding for public health.

• • •

Cape Breton is an island, and like most rural or remote places I've worked, there is a strong sense of identity. Centuries of shared history unite most of the island—in recent years there has been far more out-migration than immigration, so those who have roots here are more common than those who "come from away," as is said locally. Yet over time the island has exuded a global reach; many came from other provinces and countries, lured by resource-based industries, such as coal and steel. Now mines have closed and finding employment is often an impossible struggle. The once-hulking steel plant in the middle of Sydney eventually resulted in the infamous blight of the Sydney Tar Ponds. I began my tenure as MOH by seeing the end of that era, as the previous tar ponds site was unveiled as a stunning park and recreation area.

There are pockets of ethnic diversity throughout the island. Apart from the original Mi'kmaq peoples, all are immigrants, many with Scottish, Acadian, Irish, and English history. The neighbourhood of Whitney Pier was recently recognized as a Canadian heritage site for its rich diversity. However, as I present to council, I believe my son and I are the only dark-skinned people in the room. Council is predominantly made up of older, white-skinned men, and only two white-skinned women. The demographics of rural locations where I've worked have tended to be similar, at least in the non-Indigenous areas.

The island is separated from the mainland by a bridge, the Canso Causeway. The causeway curves gently away from the mainland, and there is both a physical and emotional sense of separation as you pass over the animated water of the Strait of Canso, which flows northwest from the Atlantic Ocean to the Northumberland Strait. From the causeway you can see the burgeoning highlands in the distance.

Crossing the causeway, with its worn "Welcome to Cape Breton" sign, is my marker of arriving home, despite there still being two hours to drive. I have had other markers in other rural settings. I have felt at home here in Cape Breton over the past year and a half, strangely at home, given my typical restlessness.

Standing in front of council, I know most of the councillors, just as I know the councillors of the other two municipalities that the health authority catchment area covers. It has been one of my goals to meet the local politicians and know local issues. Provincial- and federal-level politics, although vital and influential, can seem distant from daily life. Local work and local politics is tangible; people grasp the specifics of a policy that impacts them directly rather than through numerous tiers.

This breastfeeding initiative is one of those policies. At the health authority, a decision was made to dedicate a full-time staff person to this work. Although the MOH is often the spokesperson for public health, hard-working staff is essential to any campaign. Cape Breton has one of the lowest rates of breastfeeding initiation in the province, among the lowest in the country, and work is being done in many areas to try to address that. From tackling the availability of formula in hospitals, to having businesses sign on to a campaign to have their establishments be baby-friendly, to councils creating baby-friendly spaces, there are changes happening, slowly but definitively. This long-term outlook is the nature of public health.

I can't keep speaking with Kail crawling over my head, so I put him down and he runs into the centre of the chamber. If anyone is watching the council proceedings on television, they may wonder at the curly head running across their screen. A colleague collects Kail as he runs by. He sits in the chair beside her, still talking, but at least no longer in motion. I can focus on my messages now, then hand it over to a public health nurse who will complete the presentation with our policy recommendations.

The only comments come from the two female councillors. They applaud the initiative and relate personal struggles when breastfeeding their children decades ago. The men are silent, but they vote with the motion to support the policies we've recommended.

I gather my belongings and take Kail's hand. He sings as we make our way out of the chambers with other public health staff.

This is a public health victory: a change in policy. Steps like this, ones that involve multiple agencies, relationship building, trust, planning, and communication, are ones that motivate me as a public health physician. Public health is work that drives me daily, that gives me a sense of purpose beyond the immediate. It is work that means looking past the illness in the patient in front of me to the environment in which that patient lives, works, and plays. It is work that allows me to integrate my son in a way that shows him that health is about connections with community—even if that means having a toy truck on my head while presenting to council.

# Dr. Peter Loveridge

*Peter Loveridge is a rural doctor who has lived in Nova Scotia for over forty years. After learning to sail on the challenging east coast of England, he has been in and out of virtually every inlet and creek on the Atlantic coast of the province, always in a small boat, and often without fancy instruments. As he approaches senior citizen status, he is grateful that he now does have all the fancy stuff. Enlightenment came passing underneath one of the Halifax bridges and not being able to see the bridge deck. He remains cheerfully unrepentant about being politically incorrect and expressing his opinions as he sees things.*

## Puss in Boot

I came to Nova Scotia in November 1974.

I have been here ever since.

It was quite a transition.

I came from a rural area in the west of England. But in rural England, there is a village every ten kilometres or so, and you are never more than thirty kilometres from a fair-sized town. Here, in my home in rural Nova Scotia, the nearest town of any size is

Halifax, and that is three hundred kilometres away. In the 1970s, that meant an arduous five-hour trek. It isn't much better now.

Adjusting to the weather was also a challenge. In England's West Country, at least at sea level, snow is a once-in-every-five-years event, and there may be two or three days a year where the temperature goes below freezing. While western Nova Scotia has the mildest climate in eastern Canada, snow is not an infrequent event, and there are things like freezing rain, which I had never seen before.

So it came to pass that about three months after I took up residence, on a Saturday night in the middle of a snowstorm, I got a call from one of my neighbours. Now, unlike in England, where you could live next door to someone for a decade and never say more than "good morning" to them, all my neighbours had been very helpful in helping us acclimatize to our new environment, so I was glad to return any kindness.

"Do you think you could come over for a few minutes?" he asked.

Thinking it was a medical thing, I replied, "Sure, what seems to be the problem?"

"Ah…ah…well, the cat's got a hook in his back paw, and there's not a chance in hell we can get him to the vet in this weather."

Well, I thought it couldn't be that difficult, so I gathered my house-call bag and went across the road.

Entering the house, I was greeted by my neighbour, a high-line fisherman who at that time was making five times as much money as any of us. He looked at my bag and then said, "Don't think you'll need that, Doc, we got all the tools you need." We advanced on the cat, a huge ginger tom occupying a corner of the room, who was not in good humour at all, with much mewling, hissing, and baring of teeth. With any close approach, the claws came out, and it was clear more than just the cat would need attention with any further decrease in proximity.

"How the hell are we going to get at the beast?" I asked.

"Don't worry about that, Doc, we have a plan." My neighbour had put on thigh-high sea boots, oilskins, and thick gloves. His son, a teenager, appeared with a large pair of pliers, a set of bolt cutters, and a large boot. "Your tools, Doc," he said.

I was still mystified about how we were going to immobilize this fearsome, angry beast, but I was soon enlightened. My neighbour approached the cat, and as it tried to get past, he grabbed it.

I had wondered what the protective gear was for, and now I knew. The son, by this time, had the boot close by, and moggie was stuffed, unceremoniously, headfirst into it. There was a hell of a lot of noise, but only the two back paws were exposed and they couldn't move much.

I looked at the hook, now the first time I had seen it. Now there's hooks, and then there's hooks. This was a cod or halibut hook, and it was stuck behind what would be the Achilles tendon on a human. Now for y'all lubberly types that don't know what one of these things is, let me explain. The hook is about fifteen centimetres long and made of a rod about six millimetres thick. The round bit with the barb on it is about five centimetres in diameter, and the barb itself is two centimetres long and a centimetre wide. "He was chasing mice in the barn" was the explanation.

I realized my effete little forceps and stuff were not up to the task, and there was no chance of using the rubber-band trick to get this out. I could feel the point of the barb and, with some effort using the pliers, and much annoyance on the part of the beast, I pushed it through the skin. The bolt cutters disposed of the barb and it was then easy to back the rest of the hook out. The boot was upended and one very angry cat was shaken out. He slunk off to the basement, his usual abode, and we had a few drinks. A week or so later he was back to his usual grumpy self.

We didn't bother with antibiotics or tetanus shots, and as far as I know, he lived to a ripe old age for a rural outdoor cat. I guess I have as well.

# Dr. Mythri Kappagantula

*Mythri Kappagantula studied anatomy and cell biology at McGill University, as well as English, Sanskrit, philosophy, and music. She attended medical school at University College Dublin in Ireland, where she worked as an intern for one year before joining the Dalhousie University family medicine residency program in Fredericton, New Brunswick. She then practised in Nova Scotia in a collaborative emergency centre, a combination of a primary care clinic and rural ER. New Brunswick gave her a wonderful residency experience and she enjoyed sailing on the Saint John River. In Nova Scotia, she enjoyed snowshoeing, cottage life on the Gulf Shore, and kayaking in the Northumberland Strait. The people she encountered in the Maritimes, whether coworkers, patients, or friends, were unforgettable in their warmth and sincerity. After a long and winding journey, she loves being back home in Ottawa, where she returned to take the reins of her mother's family practice.*

## Dental Floss and Good Teeth

The road between the Trans-Canada Highway and Summervale was marked by maple tree farms, where you could stop for

delicious syrup in the spring, brightly coloured houses, and potholes reminiscent of the craters on the surface of the moon. I
always remembered to look up from the obstacle course beneath
my poor tires before I reached the outskirts of the town, when
the road suddenly came upon a view of a lake surrounded by
trees. It was equally beautiful at all times of the day, and a breath
of fresh country air welcomed me before I prepared myself for
the day ahead at the Summervale hospital. The hospital itself
stood atop a windy hill, not ideally situated for the helicopter
landing pad used by the occasional LifeFlight chopper. But it
was the perfect vantage point for breathtaking views across the
Nova Scotia countryside while patients waited to be seen at the
doctor's office.

Summervale was notable for its long history of coal mining
and the associated disasters that eventually shut down the mines
forty years ago. As a result, many of its inhabitants were of that
stoically jolly generation that spent more time underground
than above it. One of Canada's most famous musical luminaries
hailed from Summervale, and there was also a federal prison
that served as shelter and employment for large numbers of
people. Summervale was a microcosm of semi-rural Canadian
life in the Maritimes and offered me both medical and socio-
logical lessons in equal measure.

The hospital served as a family practice clinic, emergency
room, holding area for the nearby nursing homes, and much more
to the surrounding community. In truth, a trip to the hospital
was often the highlight of a person's day, and what was observed
and heard there would invariably be discussed at the local Tim
Hortons the following day. I would not say that everyone knew
everyone, but a game of Six Degrees of Separation would have
done well in Summervale. As I "came from away"—or CFA as
the Maritimers put it—I relied on the nurses and secretaries to
fill me in on my patients' backgrounds as they came through the
door. Needless to say, what I did not know about my patients'

lives when I started working in Summervale could have filled more hard drive space than all the electronic medical records in the country.

As a family doctor, I worked in the clinic and the ER, as well as caring for the in-patients recovering from hip fractures or waiting for a nursing home bed, or the palliative patients waiting for that final journey into the next realm. All of these settings overlapped, and the relationships I developed with everyone who worked in the hospital buoyed me during the insanely busy or frustrating times. When the days were filled with malfunctioning bodies and minds, the only thing that carries people through is a sense of humour, and we had more than enough laughter when I worked in Summervale.

The ER received telephone calls and in-person visits that covered issues ranging from the usual—heart attacks, strokes, fractures, pneumonias—to the more unexpected. Many of these unusual cases came through the phone, probably because people were a bit sheepish to show their faces. I will never forget when one of the ER nurses responded to a call from a fourteen-year-old whose friend had applied papier mâché around her arm and after it dried found that they had created an unexpectedly effective cast that would not come off despite their best efforts. The call on our end went something like this: "Yes, it is safe to cut it off with scissors…no you do not need to come to the emergency room to remove it…you could also just use water to dissolve the plaster again. And tell me, where exactly is your mother?" I could tell that this particular nurse had dealt with the antics of her own children by the tone of her voice.

Another memorable call that came through the ER was on the eve of the shift from daylight savings time in the spring. A very confused lady told the nurse on duty, "I have an appointment on Monday morning at 9 a.m. But because of the time change, does that mean that my appointment is really at 8 a.m.? I want to know if I need to wake up earlier to get there on time."

It was always gratifying to those of us working in the hospital that people saw the emergency room as a sort of almanac for answers to almost any question. One amateur chef even had the resourcefulness to call and ask how to cook a turkey dinner! As a vegetarian, I would have directed the "patient" to *wikiHow*, but the knowledgeable nurse explained the whole multi-step process. We thought that particular case could be categorized under "preventative medicine," since her guests were spared from an unhappy bout of Thanksgiving gastroenteritis.

One of the most meaningful memories from my time in the Summervale ER was a day when a ninety-one-year-old lady was brought in after taking a nasty tumble. She had fallen on an outstretched left hand and likely fractured some of the bones, and the swelling was already setting in. Before taking an X-ray and applying a cast, I needed to remove her wedding ring, but her finger was already very swollen. I remember the nurse working with me that shift. Her name was Julie and she possessed that indispensable combination of compassion, humour, and the ability to problem solve in a pinch. Between the two of us we were determined to remove that ring in one piece and avoid using the ring-cutter—a small but deadly device used in the management of uncooperative jewellery. We ended up improvising with dental floss wrapped around the patient's ring finger to compress the swelling, and with petroleum jelly as lubrication and some brave teeth-gritting on the part of the patient, we were successful in removing the ring. Anyone who works in health care has probably heard of the trendy term "collaborative care." For Julie and me, seeing our patient's face when we handed her the intact wedding band she had worn for over sixty years, well, that was our most rewarding collaborative moment in the ER for a long time.

On another wintry ER shift, a chatty, eighty-six-year-old gentleman with a cane came through the doors. He kept the triage nurse occupied for about thirty minutes, and I could tell that he was enjoying the social side of his visit as much as he was looking for medical help for his leg pain. When I called him into my office, he sat down with the air of someone about to tell a story. He proceeded to regale me with the tale of how he met his wife of almost seventy years, who had sadly passed away a year ago. It was evident from the way he spoke that he missed her terribly and was quite lonely without her. Another particularity of the East Coast is that your real name and your nickname are likely to be entirely unrelated. In this case, his real name was Jonathan, but he was always called Bud.

Bud told me that he met his wife when she was only sixteen and he was seventeen, and they fell in love soon after he took her ice skating. When they went to her parents to ask permission to marry, her parents refused, as they thought their daughter was too young to marry. So they continued to date for about a year, at which point Bud told me that she became pregnant. He opened his eyes wide with hands outstretched, palms up, shrugging his shoulders: "I tell you, I have no idea how that happened!" I gave him a look to say that I was onto him and he winked at me. So the couple married and raised three children. He credited his wife with everything good in their lives, praising her as a wife, mother, and person. He started to look wistful and gazed off into the distance, and I was trying to think of a way to cheer him up, when his eyes narrowed and he stared right at me.

"You married? Where are you from?"

When I told him I was unmarried, and from Ottawa, he looked at me again. "Well, I can tell you take care of yourself. And you got good teeth. You deserve a handsome man, Doc." I told Bud that I agreed with him wholeheartedly and would always remember his words of advice when the time came.

As a young female doctor of East Indian origin, the reactions of patients when they first saw me enter the examination room were variable but mostly positive. Most questioned my age, many were openly relieved I spoke English, and the majority were curious about how I landed in rural Nova Scotia to practise medicine. I did not find the personal questions invasive because that kind of inquisitiveness defines the Maritimes—people wanted to know how long I might stick around, so of course they would want to know if I was single, where I was headed next, and what they could do to entice me to stay.

Although I chose to leave to be closer to family and the place I call home—something that all my patients understood and supported—I realized that starting off as a freshly minted doctor in Nova Scotia redefined my idea of what it is to practise medicine. I learned the value of being a true generalist, of connecting to the stories and the personalities of my patients, how to crack jokes with people whose lives are so different from mine, and how to get them on board with the idea of improving their health by relating to them as human beings.

Ultimately, practicing medicine in a small community gives you the priceless gift of that feeling that you truly made a real difference in people's lives. In addition, Maritimers are as generous with their appreciation as they are with their baked goods at Christmastime and attempts at matchmaking. I know I will be back to Nova Scotia not only for a vacation but to revisit that unforgettable and formative time in the first two years after residency when the world was new and very daunting; when I just began to grasp the small but potentially powerful role I could play in the lives of the people of our beautiful country.

# Dr. Kate MacKeracher

*Kate MacKeracher recently completed her family medicine residency at Memorial University of Newfoundland and Labrador. She can drive a snowmobile, paddle a canoe, pick and preserve berries, and bake her own bread. At a young age she was once awarded a prize for building a winter shelter out of pine boughs and snare wire. She is an avid opera aficionado and is especially fond of Wagner and Massenet.*

## Between Deliveries

It was a classic "no one wins" political decision. Two thriving rural hospitals closed down to make way for a new, expensive, state-of-the-art regional hospital. The new facility was built with scrupulous fairness midway along the Trans-Canada between the two towns—in a clearing in the woods. Accessibility was excellent for the local deer population; the nearest human beings, however, faced a forty-minute round trip on a four-lane highway to reach their hospital.

As anyone but a distant politician might predict, the less-than-convenient location drove family doctors out of hospital work. The golden rural GPs, who used the gaps in their busy office practices to deliver a baby, set a broken bone, or ease the suffering of a palliative patient in hospital, became an extinct species overnight. Suddenly, there was a need for hospitalists, dedicated emergency medicine doctors, and expensive, in-house, obstetrical care. Continuity of care was decidedly thrown out with the bathwater.

Last, and least, of these troubles was the difficulty of housing trainee physicians—people who need constant timely access to the hospital for emergencies and precipitous deliveries. An efficient administrator, a relative perhaps of the politician with a penchant for boreal health care delivery, settled on the most obvious and cost-effective solution: the shiny new, but by no means luxurious, hospital call rooms.

This was how, during my PGY1 (postgraduate year 1) obstetrical rotation, the phrase, "I live in the call room," came to take on a whole new literal kind of meaning for me. A small concrete room, plus private concrete bathroom, became home for eight weeks. My nine preceptors took turns sleeping in the room next door. We shared a common kitchen and living room with emergency docs, hospitalists, visiting ultrasound techs, med students, and a variety of folks whose designation I never quite learned.

From mid-November till mid-January, I had the advantage of rolling out of bed, changing out of yesterday's scrubs into a new set, and strolling upstairs to my prenatal clinic. On several occasions, I found myself hustling to a midnight delivery still wearing my bedroom slippers. My boots started to collect dust—the ice and snow of winter in New Brunswick didn't inconvenience me in the slightest. A week or so could easily slip by before I so much as stepped out of the hospital. I started taking vitamin D tablets religiously.

I fell a bit out of contact with the outer world. The thin wall dividing my bedroom from the call room my preceptors rotated through was by no means soundproofed. Telephone conversations were necessarily public affairs. Once someone tried to mail me a letter, addressing it to "Dr MacKeracher, The Call Room, Hospital, New Brunswick." Turns out Canada Post lacks the dedication of Hogwarts's owls—unlike the letter addressed to "The Cupboard Under the Stairs," my post never arrived.

In compensation, the world within the hospital's walls became comfortably familiar. The obstetric nurses chatted with me during slow night shifts and fed me their Christmas candy. The kindly, late-night, security guards became my good friends after I repeatedly managed to lock myself out of my home/call room. The kitchen staff, tipped off by a phone call from my mom, presented me with a cake on my birthday. I had philosophical 4 a.m. conversations with my various attending staff and roomies. The assorted hospitalists and emergency doctors gradually got used to the live-in resident traipsing around their common room in her appalling green slippers and worn-out sweatpants. They looked on bemusedly as I burnt spaghetti sauce, exploded things in the microwave, and baked bread between deliveries.

One Saturday afternoon towards the end of my rotation, I girded my loins and left the hospital. I took the Trans-Canada through the winter woods to the community that used to house a hospital. Driving along the picturesque, snow-covered river, I gazed with surprised admiration at the graceful old wooden homes. I strolled the old-fashioned downtown street with its ornate brickwork buildings, browsing at the bookstore and paying a visit to the market. In fact, it was a perfectly charming country town—the sort of place I'd like to settle down in and grow roots.

Until that little field trip, however, the thought of staying in that part of the world had not even paid a fleeting visit to my mind. The medicine was great and the hospital staff were starting to feel uncannily like family, but I had no sense of place, no connection to a world outside the concrete walls and fluorescent lighting of my workplace-cum-living space, no possibility of perceiving a potential home.

For so many reasons, hospitals belong in a community, not by the side of a highway.

# Dr. Danit Fischtein

*Danit Fischtein is a mother of two beautiful children. Born in Israel and raised in Canada, she became a paramedic in Florida after high school. She then completed a nursing degree and worked as the quality and nursing manager in home care for many years in Ontario. Completing medical school in England, and clerkship in the United States and Canada, she was able to explore medicine in various parts of the world. Her residency was completed in New Brunswick, where she specialized in family medicine and emergency medicine in rural areas. Serving as a board member of Canadian Doctors for Medicare, she was able to take part in efforts to educate and improve the medicare system in Canada. Danit's interests outside of medicine include rescuing and caring for animals, travelling, boating, and water sports.*

## Big and Small

Growing up in the large, multicultural, and diverse city of Toronto gave me a mindset that did not initially prepare me for the move to New Brunswick. It was a culture shock for me to see that the population consisted of mostly white Christians, that retail stores like Walmart were not allowed to open before noon on Sundays because it was church time, that hairdressers were not allowed to open on Sundays at all, and that abortion and LGBT issues were forbidden topics of conversation.

On my first day in a family practice setting, I had a simple case with a pediatric patient. She presented with a rash that was congruent with signs of an allergy. In my mind, I knew exactly how I could help her. In addition to the usual treatment modalities, I wanted to send her to a pediatric allergist, so we could identify the source of the hives and avoid it. The staff physician (born and raised in New Brunswick) laughed at my suggestion and calmly said, "You are not in Big City Toronto anymore." As time taught me, an allergist was hard to find in the city of Fredericton, and there were no pediatric allergists in the community. It also taught me that as a physician, relying on super-specialists for every single variant was not an option. It was my job to think outside of the box, use what little resources were available, and creatively but efficiently and effectively help patients who relied on me for their health care needs.

On the flipside, when I first moved to New Brunswick, I recall asking for a pediatrician for my son. The reply I got was, "Why? What issues does your son have?" My son was a healthy three-and-a-half-year-old boy with mild asthma. At the time, he had no acute issues. I was confused. In Toronto, everyone has a pediatrician for primary care. If my son had strep, an ear infection, or needed immunizations, we saw the pediatrician within a day or two. Little did I realize that in New Brunswick, pediatricians did *not* do primary care. It is a specialist service that only deals with specific complex issues, is referral-based, offers hour-long appointments, and once the specific issue is dealt with, continuity of care is complete and the family physician resumes care. It took a while to understand all the differences seen in a rural setting, both as a patient and as a physician. Over the course of two years, I learned what the practices, expectations, and available resources are in New Brunswick.

While medicine is the same everywhere, the methodology varies greatly. Even the simplest task of ordering blood work initially seemed so complex. If someone required blood work, it was only done at the hospital. I would order blood work, and then the hospital scheduling system would book the patient for an appointment and send a letter in the mail. On the booked date, the patient would come to the hospital and take a number to wait for their turn. The wait is often an hour or more. The blood lab is always very busy and unavailable for outpatients on weekends and after 3 or 4 p.m. It also takes weeks to get an appointment at the lab. It is so different compared to Toronto, where there are private labs on every corner that are open on weekends, offer individual appointments (with no wait time), and accept walk-in patients as well. Some doctors even have labs in their buildings, specifically for them. And it is all covered by medicare, despite being private. I learned there is one private lab in Fredericton on the north side, and there is very little wait, but they charge patients extra. It is useful for those who are willing to pay but not feasible for those who need it and cannot justify the extra cost, creating inequality in health. It also goes against my principles and belief in sustainable medicare and the Canada Health Act.

Over time, I learned the appropriateness of sending people over to the hospital for urgent, same-day blood work, ECGs, ultrasounds, and X-rays. I continue to learn what is appropriate and what is not. Through trial and error, I learned which tests could be ordered urgently, how to access them, what times they were available, and how to bypass the usual methods for those that needed it sooner. I also learned that I could book diabetics (among people with other conditions) in advance every three to four months for a full year to ensure proper care. This was even extended to the emergency department, where I could write orders and send someone directly for care I could not provide in the office, without affecting the emergency physicians' patient line-up. This was actually quite a great benefit in a rural setting, which I appreciated. In a larger city like Toronto, if the primary care practitioner or pediatrician sees a patient in the community, the best they can offer is to send them to the emergency department equipped with a note or phone call from the physician, which most of the time proves to be useless.

Fredericton, although defined by many as rural, is actually not. There is a large hospital offering most services and specialists, as well as access to specialty services outside of the city if not available locally. I also work in real rural areas in New Brunswick and see bigger differences. Working with a home-visiting doctor for palliative care and at a rural community health centre in Minto (an urgent care clinic that lost funding as a hospital many years ago) is quite enlightening. There are only a few physicians in places like Minto and patient-physician boundaries are often blurred. In such small communities, the physician is well known. I spoke with several local doctors, who stated that living and working in the same place was quite problematic. Members of the community have their home phone numbers and would often call to discuss health issues at all hours of the night. Where larger centres have call schedules and a physician is "off" when not on call, a lot of rural physicians felt they were always on call. This was extremely problematic when they were at the local supermarket, or at a local community event, or having their family's Thanksgiving dinner. Several physicians find this kind of access very frustrating and many have moved elsewhere for this reason.

Resources are scarce in real rural communities. As I realized during home visits, having blood drawn from a home care nurse means that the patient or patient's family are responsible to get the blood to the lab. The closest lab was at the hospital, usually an hour or more away. I feel this is very inefficient and likely quite costly and difficult for the patient. Why have a nurse draw blood at home, when you have to take it to the hospital yourself anyhow? Even the urgent care clinic in Minto does not have lab services. Any blood drawn at the lab is sent via taxi to the hospital in Fredericton. I cannot imagine how this saves money in the bigger picture, or helps that patient who comes in with a heart attack, which is not identified until hours later (or the next day, since the clinic closes at 5 p.m.). They do have an X-ray machine in Minto, which is entered into the computer system and read by the radiologist in Fredericton. Knowing that one person is reading all of the radiology reports in such a large catchment area (in the "hot seat" at the hospital) makes me feel that we might be overwhelming that department.

These truly rural areas are deficient in choices, even to improve lifestyle. There is only one supermarket and the prices tend to be fixed. Patients are lucky if there is a pharmacy in the area, but most do not offer compounding of medications. Short supplies of medications are seen often as well, meaning a different formula needs to be used that has a shorter shelf life and higher cost to the patient. Access to organized physical activities for children is nonexistent. However, living in a rural community often means farm work and physical labour, so maybe playing soccer or T-ball is not on the top of the priority list.

Fredericton, being a small city but not as rural as other parts of New Brunswick, has many benefits that bigger cities do not experience. The fact that its hospital is family medicine-based means that most in-patients, including newborns, are followed by their family physician. This offers great continuity of care, comfort for the patients, and easier access to services in the hospital. For example, physicians can write orders and admit directly from their clinic to the hospital. They also have access to specialist referral services within the hospital, and can draw on their expertise when necessary. The nice thing in a smaller community is that physicians know each other well. If they need advice in an outpatient setting, or if they are concerned that a patient needs to be seen quicker, they can just make a simple phone call. Unlike in larger cities, a phone call does not consist of pleading and convincing the specialist that it is important that the patient needs to be seen urgently. Patient care is more efficient in that sense, and those at high risk have very quick access to care. With the incoming centralized computer systems, everything is coordinated. All specialist referrals, blood work, radiology, microbiology, and emergency visits are handled on one computer system in New Brunswick.. Every physician in the community has access to records in the entire province. Duplication is often avoided, follow-up testing is easier to recall, and knowledge of the patient's medical history is at most practitioners' fingertips. This is much more difficult to accomplish in a larger city, where large teaching hospitals across the street from each other have entirely different computer systems and record-keeping methods. It was faster to walk to the hospital across the street to print records than to access the information electronically. There is discussion that in the near future, even prescriptions and referrals will be sent out electronically and confirmations will be received through the same system.

Larger cities rely heavily on specialists and super-specialists (those who have completed several fellowships after residency and are super-experts in very defined areas of medicine) because there are so many. This reminds me of a friend who saw her family physician for dizziness in Toronto. After being diagnosed with benign paroxysmal positional vertigo (BPPV), she asked her physician if she could do the Epley maneuver to help with symptoms. The reply was that she would be referred to an ear, nose, and throat specialist for this. The Epley maneuver takes a few minutes and requires no additional apparatus aside from an examining table. I was very surprised this would require a referral, as in Fredericton this procedure is done quite often in the office by the family physician. It seemed like a waste of time and expertise—it may take months to see a specialist.

Overall, working in a rural community has both advantages and disadvantages for both the physician and for patient care.

While the pillars of the Canada Health Act exist, they do not serve true for every community. However, physicians in smaller communities and rural areas become very well-rounded clinicians who must know how to do many procedures and determine diagnoses and treatments that those in a large city may not learn or need to do. With such few specialist services and fancy diagnostic modalities, the family physician must be better equipped to ensure good-quality patient care. Many have asked me (often in shock and dismay) why I chose to move from Toronto to Fredericton. What they don't realize is that while resources may be scarcer, and while frustration with the system is common when trying to make the best decisions for patients, there is a closer community, more centralized access to care, and a greater reliance on family physicians—all of which have made me a better doctor. I hope that over time, deficiencies improve in rural settings and resources become more available for everyone, in a manner that is cost-effective and efficient. Simple things like fluoride in the water, education systems that teach preschoolers to read and write, and cheaper "healthy" foods would make smaller communities like Fredericton thrive.

But small changes *are* being made. Walmart now opens whenever it wants (as do other stores), even during church services. The blood lab in the hospital implemented new methods to improve wait times. There is a new clinic that treats transgender patients openly. And while abortion is still a hot topic, these procedures are being performed and taught in silence. Rural communities need better incentives, knowledgeable physicians, and open-minded individuals to grow, because the status quo has never led to anything special.

# Dr. Danie Ty

*Danie Ty is a firm believer in social justice and universal access to health care. She works primarily with rural, remote, and marginalized communities in North America and Southeast Asia. Originally from Montreal, she is one of five children of Khmer Rouge genocide survivors. As a result, she was raised with a healthy dose of humility, altruism, and dedication to hard work. Growing up in a single-income family with meager means, she understands the meaning of affordable quality health care for all.*

## I Am Not a Cowboy Doctor

It was the middle of the night and I was answering the phone before I even knew I was awake. I was on call and there was nothing but bad news. I had an emergency on my hands.

I looked out the window. I could barely see the thermometer perched on the sill on the other side of the pane. The raging snowstorm made it nearly impossible to read: -46°C. My heart sank. I hurriedly put on my winter gear: wool under layers, snow pants, boots, mitts, and parka. As I stood in the doorway, I squeezed my head into my neoprene balaclava and adjusted my snow goggles over my eyes. Not a bit of skin was exposed—frostbitten once and twice shy, I supposed. The hospital was less than five hundred metres away, yet the only sign of its existence in this snowy haze was a singular glowing light over its main entrance. I started on my slow and steady march towards my trusty beacon.

The ward nurse on call greeted me on my arrival and asked the reason for my midnight visit. I had been contacted via phone in regards to an older gentleman, who was in respiratory distress after receiving a blow to his left rib cage during an alcohol-fuelled bar fight. She looked around stunned and quickly peered over my shoulder at the empty resuscitation room and ambulance bay. She was puzzled as there was no one matching that description in the entire hospital. It would all seem so simple, except for a few not so minor details. I was in the North. More specifically, I was just six degrees of latitude shy of being in the Arctic Circle and isolated from all the trimmings and consultants one would find in a typical emergency department in a major city. Furthermore, the nurse who had called me was nowhere to be found. In fact, she was alone in an Inuit community three towns away, which was accessible only by plane. And the patient? He was deteriorating with every passing minute. The choice was made before I had even left my trailer apartment: the patient had to be retrieved and returned to our base hospital for treatment.

The ward nurse leapt to her feet at the mention of an emergency air evacuation and she began to make the necessary phone calls. Soon the ward radio crackled to life with familiar voices. The pilot was contacting his co-pilot. The airport confirmed that the King Air, our smallest plane, was being readied. The community driver confirmed that he would pick me up at the hospital to bring me to the airport. My colleague, another physician, was on her way. An ICU-trained nurse was already on his snowmobile racing towards the hospital. We would all fly together. Amid the chaos, I stood quietly in the supply room gathering my thoughts. I had to be methodical and selective, as I did not have the luxury of loading the aircraft with non-essential medical equipment given the limited space. The King Air was a seven-passenger plane, on which our base crew would take five seats. In order to fit a supine patient on a stretcher, the nurse, the other physician, and myself would have to sit in a row, each behind the other with the patient laid alongside us. In the unfortunate case of resuscitation, the person at the front would have to manage the airway, while the middle person would manage chest compressions and the last person would manage lines, drugs, and medications. Anyway, to further compound the difficulty of the situation, the choice of supplies was limited by the weight of the equipment that I would personally have to help carry and by my familiarity and comfort with each one. It was indeed a game of Tetris and not an easy one at that.

Soon I found myself crammed uncomfortably in the King Air alongside my colleague, the ICU nurse, and the pilot and co-pilot. The plane was cold and dark. We sat rubbing our hands and breathing into the collars of our coats, without power, trying to conserve as much fuel as possible. Whatever energy reserve we could muster now would mean the difference between powering life-saving equipment for our patient or flying the plane out of harm's way to safety. We sat silently shivering, each watching the storm through the windows. We watched as the snow fell violently to the left, then to the right, and back again. It was unwise to take off in the crosswinds and so we waited nervously until the winds were in our favour. The pilot stared straight ahead, hands on the controls, and no one talked. Suddenly, after twenty minutes of waiting, there was a momentary break in the wind. The engine roared itself awake, and the plane was off.

When we arrived, the patient was clutching at his non-re-breather face mask as the right side of his chest heaved desperately up and down. He smelled of contraband alcohol, likely smuggled into this dry community with the once-weekly air delivery of essential supplies. Unfortunately, alcohol-related brawls, accidents, and attempted suicides were linked to such delivery days in these villages. As I approached the patient, it was clear he had suffered a traumatic pneumothorax and would need to have a chest tube placed to re-expand his collapsed lung. A wave of momentary relief washed over me. Part of the anxiety of evacuations was the fear of not anticipating correctly or not being prepared for a given situation. Thankfully, I had packed not only a portable ultrasound to confirm the diagnosis but also a chest tube kit in the very school bag I used to wear to medical school.

With chest tube in hand, I nervously recited the ATLS (Advanced Trauma Life Support) steps for insertion aloud. The only chest tubes I had ever placed were in patients made of plastic in the artificial environment of a simulation lab. My colleagues watched in silent support, as they had as much experience as I did, if not less. The room felt hot and a clammy sweat began to crawl out of my skin. There was no one to defer the procedure to and the patient, increasingly unstable, could not be transported back in a nonpressurized plane without it. I hated myself for being anxious, for being scared. I felt like a coward, yet I had no choice. I had to trust myself. I had to trust my skill. I had to trust the medicine. I had to quiet my fear and my frustration and my ego, and act for the sake of the patient.

I put the chest tube in and he began to breathe. He was going to live. The patient was stabilized and transported back to our base hospital for care. The ride back was mostly uneventful. On our return, the first call I made was to the southern trauma centre with which our hospital centre was affiliated. As I spoke with the consulting emergency physician, I was horrified. He ridiculed me for not doing an X-ray before placing a chest tube and for not immediately transferring the patient down south to his trauma centre. Such ignorant encounters were not the norm, but they were common enough that I wasn't surprised.

Unfortunately, it would be naive for me to think that all consultants were well versed in the challenges of rural/remote medicine. I held my tongue and explained to the consultant that the community we evacuated the patient from did not have any sort of imaging facility, that the diagnosis was made clinically, and that the patient had to be evacuated via unpressurized, fixed-wing plane and thus needed a chest tube preflight. In regards to transferring the patient down south, I explained that I had to respect his wishes to stay in his community. Admittedly, I did try to convince the patient to accept a transfer to a tertiary care centre. However, the patient was steadfast in his refusal and began telling me stories of his family and their experiences with doctors. Tragically, there was a time when physicians passively watched Inuit die from a tuberculosis epidemic that raged in their many communities. According to him, nothing was done, at least not in the beginning. When the government finally moved to action, the seeds of distrust and anger were sowed among the Inuit. As per the patient, physicians played a role in the forceful separation of families against their will, sending members to sanitariums in the south without translators, without warning, and without informing them of where they were going or for what purpose. It was interesting to witness the continued distrust of the medical establishment in my patient. I wondered to myself if others felt similarly. The hour was late; it would have to be a thought for another day.

In the end, all was well once again. My patient was sleeping comfortably at the hospital. The ward nurse was back to reading her magazine at the main desk, waiting to be relieved by the oncoming morning staff. The fluorescent lights hummed monotonously throughout the empty hallways. And I was slowly slipping back into my slumber at home.

"Wow! You guys are such cowboy doctors up there!" exclaimed my friend as I recounted to him the string of events. I felt perplexed, maybe a touch offended. I was not a cowboy doctor by any means. I was not brave or irresponsibly gung-ho. I was not some sort of self-righteous vigilante operating outside the confines of the law or medicine. If anything, I believe rural and remote physicians share some common qualities not typically relegated to cowboys. They include the humility to admit our shortcomings, the wisdom to ask for help, the foresight to never act rashly, and the willingness to trust one's skills and knowledge. And most importantly, I would not want to draw any analogies between my patients and cattle.

# Dr. Baijayanta Mukhopadhyay

*Baijayanta Mukhopadhyay est un médecin de famille qui travaille au nord de l'Ontario et du Québec. Il est diplômé en médecine de l'Université McGill, et il a fait sa résidence à l'École de médecine du nord de l'Ontario. Anciennement sociologue, il est coordinateur par interim de la branche canadienne du Mouvement populaire pour la santé. Il est aussi écrivain, et adore le vélo et les chats.*

*Baijayanta Mukhopadhyay is a family physician in northern Ontario and Quebec. He completed his medical schooling at McGill University and his residency at the Northern Ontario Medical School. Formerly a sociologist, he is the interim coordinator of the Canadian wing of the People's Health Movement. He is also a writer, and he loves cycling and cats.*

## Rendez-vous avec ta carrière à 14 h, aujourd'hui

De l'avion, je constate que je ne suis plus à Montréal. Arrivé de la grande ville, l'Abitibi me semble encore plus immense. La forêt à perte de vue, et ces petites colonies de l'humanité coincées dans son étreinte. Même au mois d'août, la fraicheur du vent fait allusion à l'automne. J'attends l'arrivée de la navette à l'aéroport, cherchant dans mes bagages pour trouver un coupe-vent.

Je suis venu en Abitibi pour faire mon stage en pédiatrie. Je commence tout juste mon externat, un étudiant en médecine naïf, curieux, nerveux. Je venais de passer deux semaines à l'urgence de l'Hôpital d'enfants de Montréal, où il n'y avait aucun doute sur la présence d'enfants. Mais ici, y a-t-il des enfants dans cette contrée sauvage?

Le premier jour, je m'installe dans l'appartement à côté de l'hôpital, et je commence mes explorations de la ville—ou du village. C'est la première fois que je me trouve au nord. Je découvrirai avec le temps que le nord est un espace culturel, pas nécessairement géographique—c'est un mode de vie, une façon de faire.

Nous sommes dimanche. Je me rends à la rue principale en dix minutes de marche tranquille. Il y a beaucoup de petits magasins fermés. Je vois trois succursales de banques, mais la mienne, une banque majeure au pays, est absente. Les seuls commerces ouverts sont l'épicerie et deux bars. Devant l'un, il y a un vieillard qui s'endort debout. Devant l'autre, un groupe de jeunes autochtones rieurs. J'entre dans le supermarché. Je suis vraiment conscient de ma peau foncée, ma différence visible. Mais l'homme qui arrive aux caisses au même instant que moi me cède la place avec un sourire chaleureux. La caissière me salue avec un « Bonjour » indifférent—elle n'a pas l'air d'être inaccoutumée aux visites des habitants méridionaux.

Le lendemain, l'orientation à l'hôpital se déroule dans une ambiance cordiale. L'hôpital est plus petit que les hôpitaux que je connais au sud, et je m'oriente vite aux endroits importants pour un étudiant en médecine—les étages médicaux, la salle d'urgence, la bibliothèque, la cafétéria et le réfrigérateur où se trouvent les collations. Je suis impressionné par la tranquillité, la civilité des lieux. Les couloirs sont souvent vides, aucune des cohues folles des hôpitaux montréalais. Je vois beaucoup de personnes avec le teint foncé; la plupart des immigrants en Abitibi travaillent au domaine de la santé, semble-t-il. Dans l'ascenseur, un homme dans la soixantaine et sa femme m'accompagnent au troisième étage. « Il fait froid aujourd'hui, hein ? » me dit-il. « Tu n'y es sûrement pas habitué. » Je découvrirai pendant ma formation à travers le Canada que tout nouvel arrivant dans une petite ville doit certifier la croyance populaire que le climat local est le plus froid, le plus enneigé, le plus tempétueux du pays.

Je rejoins le pédiatre de garde après mon orientation. J'ai hâte de commencer, ayant déjà lu la première partie du texte pédiatrique que j'ai apporté avec moi. Mon patron est un petit homme jovial d'origine africaine. Nous faisons la tournée de nos patients, presque exclusivement des nouveau-nés cris dont les mères sont descendues au sud de leurs villages pour l'accouchement.

Ensuite le pédiatre me dit d'aller dîner. « J'ai eu un appel d'une mère qui s'inquiète de son fils. Je lui ai donné rendez-vous pour 14h. »

« 14h quel jour ? » Ma demande est très logique dans un contexte montréalais, où l'accès aux rendez-vous médicaux nécessite une analyse de logistique très avancée.

Le pédiatre me regarde un instant, déconcerté. Il répond très lentement, comme il explique une maladie à un de ses petits patients : « 14h, aujourd'hui. »

Je ne suis plus à Montréal, c'est sûr.

Le stage en Abitibi m'ouvre les yeux sur la médecine comme je voulais la pratiquer. Il ne s'agit pas seulement d'accès aux médecins. Comme étudiant, j'ai appris à apprendre de mes patients. Il n'y avait pas souvent un collègue spécialisé pour demander une consultation. J'ai dû faire une réponse réaliste et raisonnable à tout patient devenu mien. J'ai appris à écouter mes patients, à développer un rapport non seulement avec eux, mais avec leur famille, leur contexte social.

Un bébé algonquin est admis avec une bronchiolite persistante. L'admission perdure—quatre, cinq jours. Pendant ce temps, je bâtis un rapport avec la mère, qui au début était méfiante, cynique. Les infirmières l'accusent d'aller boire le soir, d'après les appels téléphoniques de la grand-mère. Mais la mère ne semble pas être ivre lorsqu'elle est là le matin. Elle me dit qu'elle a quatre autres enfants chez elle. Elle veut savoir si la bronchiolite est contagieuse. Elle est certaine que les conditions d'habitation sur la réserve sont responsables de la maladie de son petit. Elle commence à me parler des conflits de sa nation avec les gouvernements provincial et fédéral, le manque d'électricité, de logement adéquat. Il y a quelques mois, un bébé de six mois est mort de la coqueluche.

Et voilà l'autre réalité qui m'attire au nord. A moins d'une heure de cette ville minière paisible, la réalité se cache bien à Montréal, où même Kahnawake, de l'autre bord du fleuve, semble trop lointain pour avoir pertinence à la vie quotidienne d'aujourd'hui. Mais ici, pendant mon stage, la colère provenant de ma propre impuissance devant les ravages de la pauvreté et de l'exclusion devient formatrice. Pour confronter ces inégalités qui sont les plus importantes actuellement au pays, je décide de devenir un médecin de famille qui travaille dans les régions rurales et nordiques. Oui, il y a beaucoup de peuples autochtones en ville, qui doivent eux aussi faire face aux obstacles à la santé. La pauvreté existe partout. Mais ici elle est encore plus invisible qu'à Kahnawake, loin des quartiers populaires des grandes villes canadiennes. Il faudra y consacrer énergie et passion, en solidarité avec les communautés, où les outils de la médecine familiale peuvent contribuer à la longue route vers le plein épanouissement de ces enfants.

# Appointment with Your Career at 2 p.m., Today

From the plane, I can tell I am no longer in Montreal. Arriving from the big city, Abitibi seems immense. The forest is all I see, with little colonies of humanity trapped in its embrace. Even in August, the cool wind alludes to autumn arriving. I rummage through my luggage to find a windbreaker as I await the shuttle from the airport.

I came to Abitibi for my rotation in pediatrics. I was just starting my medical school clerkship, a naive, curious, and nervous medical student. I had just spent two weeks in the emergency department at Montreal Children's Hospital, where there was no doubt about the presence of children. But here, in this vast wilderness?

I move into the apartment next to the hospital and begin my explorations of the city—or village. It is my first visit to the North. I discover with time that the North is a cultural space, not necessarily geographical—it is a lifestyle, a way of doing.

It is Sunday. The main street is a leisurely ten-minute walk away. Many small shops are closed. I see three bank branches, but mine, a major bank in the country, is absent. The only open shops are the grocery store and two bars. In front of one there is an old man who falls asleep standing up. In front of the other, a knot of jovial First Nations youth. I go into the supermarket. I am very aware of my dark skin, my visible difference. But the man who happens to serve me greets me with a warm smile. The lady at the checkout greets me with an indifferent "Good morning"—it is perhaps not unusual to see an influx of southern residents.

The next day, the orientation at the hospital is cordial. The hospital is smaller than hospitals I know in the south, and I quickly orient myself to the significant places for a medical student—medical floors, the emergency room, the library, the cafeteria, and the refrigerator where I can find snacks. I am impressed by the tranquility, the civility. The corridors are often empty, with none of the crazy crowds found in the Montreal hospitals. I see many people with dark complexions—most immigrants in Abitibi work in health care, it seems. In the elevator, a man in his sixties and his wife accompany me to the third floor. "It's cold today, eh?" he says to me. "You're probably not used to this." I have discovered during my training across Canada that any new arrival in a small town must certify the popular belief that the local climate is the coldest, snowiest, and stormiest in the country.

I meet with the pediatrician after my orientation. I cannot wait to start, having already read the first part of the pediatric text I brought with me. My boss is a little jovial man of African origin. We make rounds to our patients, almost exclusively newborns whose Cree mothers came down south from their villages to give birth.

My supervisor dismisses me for lunch. "I got a call from a mother who is worried about her son. I gave her an appointment for 2 p.m."

"2 p.m. which day?" My question is very logical in the Montreal context, where access to medical appointments requires an analysis of very advanced logistics.

The pediatrician looks at me a moment, confused. He responds very slowly, as though explaining an illness to one of his little patients: "2 p.m. today."

Not Montreal, for sure.

The rotation in Abitibi opens my eyes to medicine as I want to practise it. It is not the question of access to doctors alone. As a student, I learned to learn from my patients. There was not often a specialist colleague to request a consultation. I had to develop a realistic and reasonable response to any patient who became mine. I learned to listen to my patients to develop a relationship not only with them but with their family, their social context.

An Algonquin baby is admitted with persistent bronchiolitis. While the admission continues—for four, five days—I build a relationship with the mother, who at first was suspicious, cynical. Nurses accuse her of going drinking in the evening, according to phone calls from the grandmother. But the mother does not appear to be drunk when she is there in the mornings. She says she has four other children at home. She wants to know if bronchiolitis is contagious. She is certain that the conditions of the homes on the reserve are responsible for the illness of the child. She starts telling me about the conflicts between her nation and the provincial and federal governments, the lack of electricity, adequate housing. Recently, a baby of six months died of whooping cough.

And that is the other reality that draws me north. Within an hour of this tranquil mining town lies a reality easily overlooked in Montreal, where even Kahnawake Mohawk Territory on the other side of the river seems too distant to have relevance to everyday life. But here, during my rotation, my anger at my own helplessness before the ravages of poverty and exclusion becomes a focal point. To confront these inequalities that are currently the most significant in the country, I decided to become a family physician who works in rural and northern areas. Yes, there are many Indigenous people in cities who must also deal with health barriers. Poverty exists everywhere. But here, far from the teeming neighbourhoods, it is even more invisible than in Kahnawake. It requires devotion, energy, and passion to work in solidarity with communities, where the tools of family medicine can contribute to the journey towards realizing the full potential of the children of the North.

**ONTARIO**

# Dr. Fahreen Dossa

*Fahreen Dossa is a rural family physician who completed a diploma in tropical medicine after graduating from the University of British Columbia's rural medicine residency program. She has worked in a number of remote communities in northern British Columbia, northern Ontario, and the Northwest Territories. She has a passion for international health and spent three years working in Afghanistan and Pakistan. She has also worked with* Médecins Sans Frontières/ Doctors Without Borders *and other nongovernmental organizations in Liberia, Nepal, and Tanzania. When she is not working in the North or overseas, she is at home with her family in Vancouver.*

## Call of the North (a.k.a. The Uninvited Guest)

I swallow the bile in my throat as the tiny, nine-seater plane lurches in the air and dips low into winter cloud once again. I don't often experience air sickness, but I've been engrossed in the inflight magazine, and reading on the bumpy flight has triggered some exquisite nausea.

"Ladies and Gentlemen, we are starting our descent. Please return your seatbacks and tray tables to the upright and locked position, and please ensure that your seatbelts are securely fastened." Our brave little plane is too tiny to boast tray tables, reclining seats, or even window shades, but protocol is not to be abandoned. As the automated announcement replays in the familiar cadence of Oji-Cree, I gaze out the tiny window at the vast expanse of land below us. Summer or winter, the endless interlacing chain of lakes never ceases to impress me. "Lakes are windows into the soul of the earth," a friend and colleague once told me, and looking down at the pristine natural beauty of the northern Canadian Shield, I can't help but agree.

The land here has always drawn me, not only for its beauty but for its vastness. I feel like I can take a deep breath up here and fill my lungs with space, clarity, peace, and time. I also feel incredibly small when I travel north, not just personally but professionally, too. Everything about the North reminds me of my own insignificance, and I appreciate the perspective.

And now in the dead of winter, when the snow-blanketed land stretches untouched for hundreds of kilometres, its endless reach merging seamlessly with the vast and overarching whiteness of sky, I feel about as big as a speck of dust. In this season, especially, our fates rest entirely on the elements. Flights are often cancelled, planes cannot land, and passengers (and patients!) are often "weathered" and unable to move in or out of home communities.

I draw in a sharp breath as we touch down unevenly on the ice-covered landing strip, thankful to have reached our destination in one piece. The forty-below air is biting as the co-pilot opens up the hatch. My Sorel boots crunch the snow outside the plane, and I look around me, feeling self-conscious in my down parka and ultra-warm footgear. Most of the folks who get off the plane with me wear running shoes.

We huddle together in the wooden, box-sized building that constitutes the airport terminal, awaiting the co-pilot and the airline agent who are busily unloading our baggage. The snow blankets everything. Hard-packed snow and ice paves the roads and the lakes as well. Ice roads are well travelled in the winter months, trucking in supplies that have to be flown in at other times of the year. I wonder if my food box has made it onto the plane. As often as not, the nurses take pity on me when it doesn't, and I have learned the hard way to pack snacks in my carry-on so I don't have to rely on the PoleStar Store.

The PoleStar Store is the only grocery store in town. It is where most if not all community members buy their food. It is where a carton of milk costs $5 and a bottle of pop costs ninety-nine cents. I wonder what I might buy if money was tight and my children were hungry and an apple cost $3.50 and a bag of chips $1.50. Fresh vegetables and fruit are hard to come by at the PoleStar. What is available is often wilted, aged, and well-travelled, not to mention prohibitively expensive. I am not alone in the belief that access to food in the North (or the lack thereof) is what has triggered the epidemic of diabetes sweeping through the communities and devastating families with disability, death, and despair.

The airline agent looks over at me, "Is that yours?" He points to a large cardboard box sealed with packing tape. My food box has arrived after all. "*Meegwetch*," I nod as I collect it gratefully and search for the driver who will take me to the clinic. I poke my head outside and ignore the icy blast of air as I scan the trucks for the Health Canada logo, hoping it isn't obscured by snow or dirt. I find it and catch the eye of the driver, Billy, who grins at me from the cab, heat running full blast. I brace against the cold, which freezes my eyelashes and turns my hair white with frost. I make a run for the truck and Billy, bless his soul, gets out of the truck to help me load up the luggage.

• • •

Late that evening at the "transient apartment" attached to the clinic, I unpack the rest of my food and, too tired to eat, crawl into bed. I've had a solid afternoon clinic, along with two emergency after-hours assessments. One, a middle-aged woman struck in the leg with a baseball bat, is unable to bear weight and has likely suffered a fracture. We splint her and treat her pain, but she requires an X-ray and needs to be medevacked (medical evacuation by air ambulance). The other is a teenager who punched a brick wall over the weekend and likely suffered a boxer's fracture. She, in turn, is treated and splinted and a schedivac (medical evacuation by scheduled commercial flight) is arranged for the next day. I fall asleep thinking about both of these patients and the events that led to their respective injuries.

Something jars me sharply out of deep sleep before midnight. It takes me a moment to figure out that it is the phone. "Hello," I mumble sleepily.

"Doc, we need you to come in right away."

"Ok, sure," I sigh, "What is it?"

"We have a teenager here who came in not breathing."

Nothing can get my feet moving more quickly. I don't ask any further questions but race to the clinic, pausing only to grab my stethoscope. The nurses are excellent. One is an ex-ICU nurse and tells me that he assisted the patient's breathing with a bag and mask on arrival and then stopped when she exhibited spontaneous and regular respirations. The other nurse quickly hands me a set of vitals as I enter the room. I eyeball the patient and glance at the vitals. A thin-looking, teenage girl lies supine on the stretcher, eyes closed as if sleeping. I see her chest rise and fall smoothly. Her colour is good and her mouth is closed. There is no stridor, no bleeding, and there are no obvious injuries or deformities. Blood pressure 110/65, HR 80, RR 12 SaO2 98 per cent on room air. I relax imperceptibly. She is cardiovascularly stable, and I have time to think things through. That's when the overpowering smell of gasoline permeates my consciousness and makes me reel.

"It's more than the usual gas sniffing," the nurses brief me quietly. "She broke into the water main and was asphyxiating herself with the gas line when the police found her. She was unconscious when they brought her here."

My patient is eighteen years old and wanting to die. My heart is lead as I perform a primary survey and a quick secondary survey. There is no physical evidence of trauma, but she is unresponsive to pain and tolerates an oral airway too well. This means she has no gag reflex and cannot protect her airway. She is at risk of aspiration and needs to be intubated.

Her chart is painfully bare: no medications, no known drug allergies, no known past medical history to speak of. I call down to our base hospital ER to let them know what is going on. I take stock of the fact that we have no actual induction agents or other intubating medications in the nursing station. We have a single 5cc vial of midazolam (a short-acting benzodiazepine amnestic).

We call the air ambulance to request a medevac. Given the weather, we don't know how many hours it will take for them to arrive.

I take a deep breath and choke again on the heavy, acrid smell of gasoline. I briefly wonder whether I should instruct all of us to wear masks so we don't pass out ourselves. The thought comes and goes while I focus entirely on the equipment we need to intubate. I haven't had a chance to check the equipment since I landed. Luckily, everything is working, including the suction and the light on the laryngoscope. I re-examine the patient and see that she is thin, almost cachectic. I ask the nurse to give her 2 mg of midazolam IV. Her temperature and blood sugar are normal. I have no idea when she would have last eaten. Her family was called when she was first brought here, but none of them have come to the nursing station.

I assess her head and neck and ask for a size 7 tube with a size 6.5 on standby. I position the laryngoscope and remind myself to "lift" rather than "lever" so as to be mindful of her teeth. I ask for some *burp* cricoid pressure from the nurses. We review this beforehand, and although neither nurse is familiar with the technique, they learn it quickly and help me to protect her airway and visualize her cords. I position the tube and quickly realize it is too large. *Darn.* I need to change to the size 6.5. The nurses are quick and I am stone-cold grateful (good nurses are more valuable than gold). We make the switch quickly. The number 6.5 tube passes easily through her cords; now the challenge will be manually assisting her breathing, as there is no automated ventilator to do the job.

I inflate the cuff, but before I tape the tube into place, I move to listen to her lungs. I have my stethoscope in my ears when she bucks and instinctively reaches for her tube. Semiconscious, she pulls it out before I can stop her. I grab the suction and pray that she doesn't go into laryngospasm. My prayers are answered—she doesn't. She is suddenly awake and thankfully breathing.

She looks up at us, blinking, bewildered, and in pain: "My throat hurts," she rasps. I wonder if she can smell the gasoline in the room. I know that the pain in her throat is at least partly from the intubation/extubation, which she will not remember due to the midazolam. I sit down beside her and explain what has happened since she was found. She tells me she remembers breaking into the plant and wanting to die. She begins to cry. She shakes her head when I ask her if she still wants to hurt herself. We talk for some time and she nods when I finally ask her if she wants to/is willing to leave the community for further counselling.

Eventually, as we care for the patient and prepare her for transfer, bits and pieces of her story come to light. Her family ostracized her for her sexual orientation. Alone, rejected by those closest to her, bereft of coping strategies or community services, she sought solace in substance abuse. Ultimately, she sought solace in death.

All in all, my patient's case is not so unique. Countless northern patients face isolation, exclusion, depression, and suicide. The statistics are both sobering and shocking. We speak of the epidemic of diabetes, but there are other epidemics at play.

Plagues of pain and exclusion, of marginalization and disempowerment, of inter- and multigenerational trauma, of depression and despair.

There is both inter- and intracultural disregard, disrespect, stereotyping, and othering. There is hopelessness, confusion, and abdication on all sides. On top of this, there is rampant lack of access to healing resources, to coping strategies, to basic infrastructure, to parenting skills, to health care, to nutrition, and to educational opportunity.

There are people with far better vision and understanding to speak to all of this than me. The challenges feel daunting, innumerable, and incapacitating.

And yet, I see Elders who lead traditional healing ceremonies with faith, courage, dignity, and grace. I see entire communities come together to build youth camps and then start suboxone programs so that people addicted to prescription drugs can take their lives back.

I see how people revere the land and honour the bounty it offers them. I see that no one builds property on waterfront or "claims" lakeshore as private land. I see how neighbours often hunt and provide for each other and for the Elders in the community who are unable to provide for themselves.

I witness a deep respect for a traditional way of life. I observe how communities have preserved and nurtured native language in daily rhythms and with it a powerful sense of culture and identity.

I see how community ties have been built. I observe how children are adored and also trusted as sources of wisdom and playfulness. I hear my patients, along with the staff at the clinic, laughing together. I behold how healing this medicine is.

I have been able to participate in sweat lodge ceremonies that evoked deep spirituality and experiential wisdom. I have felt how transformative these ceremonies can be.

I have seen how difficult it has been for some to start to live off the land again, to claim space and reclaim culture. It is hard to claim power when one has been disempowered; to claim rights and voice; to claim presence.

And yet, I have witnessed the pride and care that some individuals chose to invest in this struggle. I have observed role models emerging, and I have met people who are leaders, teachers, healers, and visionaries. I met one community member who ran a marathon and returned home to start a walking program, and another who went away to school and then came back to provide tireless nursing care in the community where she grew up.

I have seen hope that prevails beyond the boil-water advisories and externally imposed school hours. I have witnessed awareness and peace amidst neglect and injustice. I have observed deep communion with nature and the healing effects of this connection.

I will never know the pain and suffering of these people. And yet I can bear witness to hardship, adversity, and anguish, as well as to dignity, courage, and forbearance. I can sit with my patients, and I can stand in solidarity.

As a testament to the generosity of the people I worked with, I was often asked to join a feast or taken fishing or welcomed into a sweat ceremony. Me, the "expat," the foreigner in this land, the stranger who stuck out like a sore thumb in her down parka and clunky Sorels.

And I wondered: As a guest here, an expat working in a clinic whose opening hours often feel imposed on my patients' lives, have I truly been invited? If so, by whom? And invited or uninvited, am I the kind of guest who gets invited back? I do not have the answers to these questions, but I am glad to be able to ask them.

In the interim, gratitude accompanies my travel north. Thank you to my patients for trusting me with your stories. Your honesty and bravery are inspiring. You have my deepest respect for your courage and tenacity through those times when hope seems lost. I admire your innovation and strength, and I esteem your inner knowledge and all the kinds of wisdom that manifest themselves in your journeys (including the kind that allows a person to ask for help). I am grateful to many of you for your abiding sense of humour, which is joyously contagious and eases many trials.

I celebrate and honour my colleagues, without whom I could not and would not do this work. A deep bow goes to the front-line nurses, whose tireless, endless, and competent care often means the difference between life and death for those in acute emergency or who are sick and weathered up north. To the allied health professionals I sometimes have the pleasure of meeting at the nursing station—hats off for your perseverance and much needed presence. To the pharmacists and other caregivers who go above and beyond to provide service to people whose summer roads are relegated to the sky, I admire your ethic of excellence and your creativity. To my fellow physicians who have been working so hard for so long, I am in awe of your long-standing commitment and devotion, your humility, your resourcefulness, your insight, your patience, and your dogged determination and hard work. Thank you for seeing injustice and fighting the good fight. Your work fills my heart and lends wings to my feet that I may continue to work alongside you.

To really listen, I must be silent. A good friend once pointed out that the words "listen" and "silent" share the same letters. So when my patient's storied symptoms don't fit snugly into the algorithmic paradigms of my allopathic training, I will try to look again and allow space and silence for the paradigm to shift. How grateful I am to the North for the vastness of its space and the silence of its snow, through which I so clearly hear this call.

**ONTARIO**

# Dr. Clare Ward

*An international sabbatical in 2007 allowed Clare Ward to experience medicine in northern Ontario. This opportunity left her with a great respect for the rural doctors in Canada and the environment in which they practise. For the past twenty-four years, she has worked in the far north of Aotearoa (New Zealand), in Hokianga, which has a predominantly indigenous Maori population. She is based in a remote rural hospital with ten acute beds, which provides acute and emergency care, palliative care, as well as obstetrical services. Ten outlying community health clinics are also serviced from Hokianga Hospital.*

## North Ontario

There are huge distances to cover. If you were on foot, you might never get from Toronto to Moose Factory, or you would not get there this year.

By train, you pass through forests of maple and then silver birch. You see nothing but bare branches and occasional yellow leaves hanging onto the last vestiges of summer. You pass through places with unfamiliar names—North Bay, Matheson, Cochrane, Otter Rapids, Moosonee—and finally complete your journey in a small boat across the river to Moose Factory. By now, the overwhelming impression is one of distance. It is an impression that will grow as you find that half an hour north by fixed-wing plane there is a peripheral clinic and that other clinics lie further on into the distance. It is autumn and the railway track is passable, the roads are passable, the weather is clement, and aircraft can come and go. In autumn, Moose Factory is an island surrounded by the grey water of Hudson Bay, surrounded near and far by wind in the birch leaves. The roads are potholed and full of water. The sky is dull, with just a little sun on a few aged wooden houses. There are no signs to speak of, and people and dwellings are almost concealed within the natural environment.

You are met by the chief of the health service, who is Cree and who tells you there are ninety-five nations and that each has about a square mile of reservation land with almost nothing given back to them by the nation-state.

Later, you meet Peter, a dialysis patient, also Cree, who tells you he shifted here from his own place 145 kilometres away so his daughters could go to school. He talks about hunting moose—best done on windy days when noise and scent are carried away from the hunter—also of getting caribou, Canada goose, snow goose. He talks about fishing for white fish (to be smoked or flaked), pike, sturgeon, pickerel in nets, of snaring rabbits and some birds, of trapping mink, foxes, beaver, and otter. He says he has often seen black bears but has not bothered them and they have not bothered him. You realize how much had been hidden from your eyes on that long train journey. You also realize that much has been taken from the people of the land here and that colonization has again come at the cost of culture, language, health, life, and autonomy.

This will be a recurrent realization, and you encounter it again in Sioux Lookout, where you meet the grandfathers.

You are invited to participate in a sweat lodge ceremony, and one wet evening you walk three kilometres out of town to a place among white tree trunks where there is a teepee and a smaller dome-shaped tent. A fire is burning and at its centre are the grandfathers.

You enter the dome through its single flap opening and into a space without light, without sound, without direction. The guide throws something onto the hot stone ancestors and it sparkles orange for a moment. It gets hot. He talks about the grandfathers in two languages—Ojibway and English. He sings and beats a drum. After a while, the flap is opened and more grandfathers come in. It gets hotter and hotter. Sweat pours out. One by one, the women there talk about what is their main concern. It could be a sick daughter or financial difficulties or sickness. At the end of each contribution the whole group says "to all my relations and *miigwech*" (thank you).

The flap opens again. Through it you can see steam and trees, inside for a moment you see the shapes of the other ten or so people. Now the men speak.

There are four sessions. Between each one more grandfathers enter. With each addition the place becomes hotter.

Within the sweat lodge, history takes the present and makes it part of itself. Within the sweat lodge, the ancestors look after their descendants and no one is alone.

Later, we return to the big teepee and share fruit and water.

The last drop of sweat beads, and gravity returns it to earth.

Then someone gives us a lift back along the edge of Pelican Lake to Sioux Lookout.

Sioux Lookout is hospitable in every way. You see the communications centre that connects far outposts to Sioux Lookout and which represents assistance, often across hundreds of kilometres, from some small place to its nearest hospital. You also connect with First Nations people who relate to the fact that you are a New Zealander from Aotearoa, another colonized country and one that is also going through the process of reconciliation. A reconciliation of past injustices with both recognition and retribution, which is more often symbolic because the real costs either cannot be calculated or cannot be afforded. You meet Garnet, who tells you of his upbringing in a residential school—as one of the children who had been taken from his own people to go to the school. Later, we go with the director of First Nations health to Dryden to see the residential school exhibition, which turns out to be a very moving record of how an entire culture was threatened with extinction by assimilation and the process of forcibly taking children out of their homes and placing them in distant residential schools. Now, as at home in New Zealand, must come the processes of reconciliation and healing.

Always underlying medicine there is the need for healing. If you could heal the injuries visited upon peoples whose lives have been damaged by two or three centuries of actions and policies, some deliberate, some accidental, then you could also change the course of disease, which is related to loss of identity, loss of wealth, loss of culture, loss of autonomy.

There are huge distances to cover. Distances filled by maples, larches, silver birch. Distances that encompass rivers and lakes and the lives among them—that also encompass the people who came here, both First Nations and the ones who came later. Their stories of survival, then and now. Survival within nature, then and now, against elements natural and unnatural. Survival in the face of isolation and distance and the isolation that is born of cultural disruption.

Still and forever remain the land, the rocks, the grandfathers.

**ONTARIO**

# Dr. Danie Ty

*Danie Ty is a family and emergency medicine physician in Canada and the United States. She graduated on the dean's list from McGill University with a bachelor of science degree, majoring in physiology. She then went on to receive her M.D., C.M. degree from McGill University and again made the dean's list. She completed her family medicine residency at Ottawa University and a third-year emergency medicine specialization at McGill University, where she was chief resident. Danie Ty currently resides in the United States with her loving husband, Brian, and their daughter, Eloise.*

## Horse Kicks, Talking Heads, and Bear Chases—Oh My!

My day was winding down and I was quite literally wrapping up my last case in the ER. My patient, an older gentleman, had been kicked squarely in the distal femur while trying to clean his horse's stable. Not surprisingly, he had sustained a fracture. His face glowed red in silence as I casted his leg. He was a rancher through and through and he was tough. Not a word, moan, or groan passed his lips. His wife sat on a stool in the corner of the room with an air of self-satisfied delight.

"I knew it! I absolutely knew it! I knew he had a broken bone when I caught him hobbling around the farm on two by fours under each arm for crutches!" she teased him. The patient's face glowed ever redder. "And that was last week!" she cackled to herself. The patient sat sheepishly on the stretcher, clearly embarrassed that it took him so long to come into the ER. Last week? I thought to myself. My patient had been walking on a broken leg for the last week? I always had the idea that country folk were more robust than their city-slicker counterparts, but this was unbelievable. It was actually quite impressive. The cast hardened and that was the end of my shift.

As I left the emergency department, I made a mental summary of my day. Morning clinic seem to have gone well, the day shift in the ER was uneventful, and it was now time for my in-patients. I only had a few patients to see, I thought to myself. I'd be home soon. I rounded the corner and made my way down the long corridor towards the medical ward. I peeked my head into the ICU as I walked by—all the patients were sleeping, not a single beep from the monitors and the ICU nurse smiled quietly at me from her station. In the medical ward, I grabbed the charts for my three in-patients and flipped through them quickly, glancing at their respective diagnoses: congestive heart failure, pneumonia, and dementia. They were all fairly straightforward cases. I began my rounds.

My first patient—the one with congestive heart failure—was doing quite well. She was responding to her diuretic therapy. She'd be home by the end of the week. Next. My second patient—the one with pneumonia—was stable. He was neither improving nor worsening. I reviewed his cultures, verified that the appropriate antibiotics were prescribed, and decided that a tincture of time was all he needed. As I approached my last patient's room, I heard the ICU nurse call out my name. I turned around and saw her rushing down the hallway towards me. Darn, I thought sarcastically to myself. She had come to save me from a mundane evening of basic cable TV and a microwave dinner. I smiled as she approached.

"There's something wrong with Mr. Rogers, Doctor! He is not all compos mentis," said the nurse as she twirled her right index finger in a circle towards her head. I reviewed my patient roster in my mind as I followed her back to the ICU. Mr. Rogers wasn't on my list. As it turned out, I was replacing a physician who was on vacation. However, that particular physician had agreed several months beforehand to cover yet another physician's patients while that latter one was also away at a conference. And he had never mentioned it to me. Such was the life of a locum rural family physician. One would have to be Alan Turing to decode the convoluted enigma of vacation/conference/illness/family-emergency schedules of rural physicians. The nurse told me Mr. Rogers was my patient and so he was. I did not question it.

Mr. Rogers was a jolly kind of man. He was heavy-set, with bright white hair sticking out in all directions, a big belly, pink cheeks, and a thunderous laugh. He was giggling to himself as I walked in. His face was contorted into a half-smile with drool dribbling from his lips. "Is this my arm, Doctor?" he gurgled, as he tried to pick up his flaccid right arm with his left hand. Santa Claus seemed to be having hemiparesis. After a quick set of vitals and a capillary blood glucose test, it was becoming evident that Mr. Rogers was having a stroke. The nurse and I grabbed the side rails of his stretcher and whisked him away to the scanner for a head CT.

Refresh. Nothing. Refresh. Nothing. Refresh. The screen paused momentarily as an hourglass appeared and there it was—Mr. Rogers's brain scan. It looked like a stroke, but not really. The colour was not as one would expect and the area of involvement was not typical for what the patient was experiencing. I did not know what to do. If I diagnosed a stroke, I might have to consider giving a thrombolytic. If I gave a thrombolytic, and there was a complication like a massive intracranial bleed, I would not be able to do very much for the patient other than palliation (make him feel comfortable). Worse, the patient was in no condition to give informed consent and we had no familial contacts with whom to discuss the matter. There were a million thoughts in my head.

Then I heard a voice: "There is definitely a sub-acute stroke. What does the patient look like?" I turned around, expecting to see one of my colleagues hovering over my shoulders. Instead, a computer on wheels greeted me with its screen facing my direction. There was a live-streaming video of the head of a man, who seemed to be sitting in some sort of office elsewhere. I looked at him in wonderment. *How long had he been there? How many times had he seen me compulsively click the refresh button on my keyboard? Why had he not made a sound sooner?* To distract me from my stream of thoughts, the head nurse gesticulated behind the wheeled computer and mouthed the words: "Tele-Health—Code Stroke." I had forgotten about the service. Tele-Health was designed to be a real-time means of telecommunication, allowing rural physicians access to distant consultants during an emergency, such as the one I was in. Suddenly, the talking head made a loud clearing of his throat and introduced himself as Dr. Nerve, the neurologist on call, based at the tertiary care centre closest to our hospital.

After the requisite introductions and case presentations, I carted my colleague towards the foot of my patient's bed. We both agreed that a neurological examination was needed, but that was easier said than done. I explained to the patient that he had to follow Dr. Nerve's instructions. However, Mr. Rogers would have none of it. He thought we were trying to make a fool of him by having him interact with what he thought was a television set. I tried to explain the concept of Tele-Health to the patient, but it was of no use. The harder I pressed, the more the patient refused to cooperate. Finally, my colleague dictated what he wanted examined, and I, in turn, faithfully executed the requested examination maneuver with my patient. My head was on a swivel as I spoke with Dr. Nerve, then the patient, then back to Dr. Nerve, then the ICU nurse, and back to the patient, and so on. I felt like I was going mad. I had a talking head dictating my every movement as if I was a marionette. Meanwhile, my patient tried to mirror my movements while demanding that his television set be shut off because the man in it was talking to us and, thus, scaring him. It was quite the scene of physical comedy.

In the end, Mr. Rogers's symptoms resolved spontaneously and Dr. Nerve was content with remotely monitoring the patient for a few days more. I packed my bag and glanced at my last in-patient. He was his usual. He was pleasantly demented in his room, talking to himself. There was nothing more to do, and so I headed home and right to bed.

It was about four in the morning when the phone rang and it was the ward nurse. "Sorry to bother you, Doctor, but I'm obliged to call you for all incidents, however small. There's been a situation with one of your patients—the one with dementia. He's perfectly fine and it's quite minor. I'll tell you about it when you come in for your morning rounds in two hours. The report will be on his chart." I hung up the phone and went back to sleep.

In the morning, I picked up all of my in-patient charts and sat down to review the overnight nursing notes. One of them had an incident report taped to the front cover. In regards to my demented patient in room 220, it read: "Patient saw bear in window. Left room and tried to leave hospital. Reason given: patient wanted to play with bear." I chuckled to myself as I signed off on the report. What a strange fantasy to have. I finished up my morning rounds and on my way out I ran into the head nurse. I asked her, "Since when did the patient in 220 start having hallucinations about bears?" She looked at me and said matter-of-factly: "Oh no, Doctor. He wasn't hallucinating. There were bears in the parking lot last night. They were probably in the trash cans looking for food. It's almost time for them to hibernate, you know. My goodness, by the time we found him, the patient made it halfway out the front door trying to get to them."

I was wide-eyed and speechless. First, I had erroneously assumed that my patient had had a psychotic break. And second, there were bears here?!

Seeing my surprise, the nurse added, "You know you're in the country now, right, Doctor?" The only words I could muster in that moment were, "I just love rural medicine."

**ONTARIO**

# Dr. Chetan Mehta

*Chetan Mehta completed his B.A. in history with a minor in math at Trent University, followed by an M.A. in history at the University of Toronto, his M.D. at McMaster University, and family medicine training at the University of Toronto. Following residency, he became addicted to working in James Bay and northern Ontario for his first year and a half in practice before returning to the city and practicing in the greater Toronto area.*

## Chasing Moose

Being a recent family medicine graduate on the reserve was exhilarating, awe-inspiring, and heart-wrenching. It's a mixture of red wine, dark chocolate, and fine cigar smoke—sweet, bitter, mildly repulsive, and intoxicating. Feelings are euphoric initially, but over time they are tempered by reality and rurality. It's Shakespearean—it is tragedy marked with comedy or, more often, comedy marked with tragedy—the only things that are different are the endings to these acts and plays. Given recent events in the news from places like Attawapiskat, Kashechewan, or other reserves and Indigenous communities, the ending is still undecided, the curtain has not yet fallen. I can still see the comedy on the horizon.

My first month in the North began with a flight from Toronto to Timmins and onwards to Moosonee in October. Prior to departure, I was stocked with Indian spices, lentils, and flour for the anticipated isolation and scarcity of vegetarian goods. As I stepped off the plane in Moosonee, I entered an airport that reminded me of a bus station in southern Ontario. While I waited patiently for my luggage to unload, two somewhat official-looking men wearing heavy rain galoshes stood outside beside a van. They were scooping up what looked like medical supplies from the plane. The North is peppered with family doctors who belong to some combination of the 3Ms—merchants, misfits, or missionaries. And this place was no exception.

"Are you the doc from Toronto here for the month?" I was asked.

"Yup."

"Well, Dr. Davidson is expecting ya—we'll stop in to see if he's at home. He's gonna orient ya around here."

We began the journey on an unpaved muddy road. Luckily, on this day, there was no following plume of dust marking our journey due to the recent rains. I was in a different Canada. To begin with, there was no pavement. There were no traffic lights. My cell phone had no reception. I definitely looked funny compared to all of the locals with my jet-black hair, dark-chocolate skin, my thoroughly Caucasian features, and my speech. I knew that the men who drove me, similar to the locals here, were used to seeing non-white, city-slicking southerners come up for work. I couldn't gauge whether being the other type of Indian—subcontinental—allowed them to feel a little closer and more connected to me, but this was not a question I would have been able to answer at the time. My sense was that trust would take time to earn, that this was not something given easily or lightly by people here, as they were used to seeing a whole slew of southerners come and go. I was ferried to a dock, where I leapt onto a motorboat, then was ferried to an island, unloaded into a van, and driven to a house where I met Dr. Davidson, who gave me an orientation to the island and my roommate, a locum dentist.

I begin with a comedic tale, a story that speaks to a world of intergenerational disconnect and how people can co-inhabit the same geographic space and yet operate in different worlds—worlds that frequently collide within hospital walls.

My first visit to a rural nursing station was wild—I cannot think of a more apt word to describe it. I had a vague inkling from what other physicians had told me, but you never know what things are really like until you're there. As I prepared throughout the week for my first visit up the coast, I was told by the hospital administration that I would need to pack food as well as my personal stuff for a four-day journey "up the road," which I kept thinking was a car ride, to my first visit on the coast. As I arrived at the airport parking lot with my cloth bags filled with prepared food to go "up the road," I immediately had to repackage all my food for the plane ride, much to the airport staff's frustration. Apparently, "up the road" included being up in the air, much to my chagrin.

And so my first trip up the coast started with a delay due to weather; too much fog for the pilots to safely land and a lot of wind. So we left an hour and a half late on the Monday. When we got on the plane, the flight up the coast was barely half an hour; it felt like the plane had simply been reparked. Raising my head as I stepped off the plane, I looked around at what felt essentially like a suburban driveway in the city but surrounded by unstoppable nature. I had this feeling for the first time, for better or worse, that I was going to be where the figurative medical buck stopped in this community and that this was the edge of civilization in this first-world country.

Quickly driven from the landing strip to the nursing station, I was scolded by the charge nurse that I was already half an hour behind for the first patient in the clinic and that the line-up had already started. Given that it was a packed clinic schedule, there was no time to dawdle.

Tossing my bags in the nearby accommodation and scarfing down a hastily assembled lunch, I got to work. As expected, the charts were thick and everyone I saw had multiple medical and psychosocial issues that couldn't be addressed on separate visits. This was complicated by the fact I didn't know these patients. I started out by running overtime by ten or so minutes on every thirty-minute appointment—thank god for the odd missed appointment! I was already in well over my head when I was suddenly pulled aside by one of the clinic nurses, who said to me, "Dr. Mehta, Dr. Peter is on the phone and would like to speak to you."

"Oh! Okay."

I took the phone and spoke to a colleague I had never met.

"Hello, is this Chetan?"

"Yes, speaking."

"I'm the emergency doctor on call at the base hospital who is fielding all of the emergency calls from up the coast. I have an emergency here and I need the help of another colleague to see this patient; the nurse seeing this patient cannot give an accurate enough description to the questions that I am asking and I cannot gauge what is happening. Would you be able to see this patient and work with me to handle what is happening there, as this situation is too serious to handle over the phone given the instability of this situation?"

"Of course, not a problem," I replied with false surety. In the meantime, I could feel the adrenaline surging and my heart starting to palpably thump as I walked over to the emergency bay at the nursing station to assess what was going on.

I promptly started asking questions of the young nurse handling the traumatic situation. "What's the patient's name? Age? Where is the chart? Tell me what the story is again?" This was a woman in her mid-fifties, who looked much older than her stated years. She was a mother to ten children, grandmother to many more, and a wildly uncontrolled diabetic on a good day and currently unconscious but breathing. A slew of family members, who ranged from being bewildered to outright sobbing, framed the chaos.

"Well, Doc, the family told me that she was unconscious on the ground and they brought her here. That was about it."

"Well, did anyone see it happen?"

"I dunno."

"Was she home alone?"

"No, the kids were there."

"Did anyone hear anything? Did she have any pain anywhere before this happened? Did she have chest pain? Did it look like she had a seizure? Did she complain of any funny speech or numbness?"

As I asked this young nurse these questions, while in parallel repeating questions to the family members, the monitors beeped occasional vital signs in my direction. Questions that were answered "yes" in one minute became "maybe" or "no" in the next. More family arrived as I tried to assemble a story with a semblance of a beginning, middle, and end.

Clues were not forthcoming. I was dumbstruck as to what the cause could be that had resulted in this peacefully unconscious woman laying before me.

My forehead was wet, the room was warm, I thought I appeared calm. It was clear to me that there was no one spokesperson appointed for making rapid decisions in what felt like an urgent situation to me. There were huddles and deliberations over everything as a clan. I felt increasingly suffocated by the lack of air movement in the room. I feared to broach the topic of end-of-life care.

On the telephone, I relayed the limited story to other ER docs in southern Ontario and their specialist counterparts, with the hope of transporting this woman safely to a larger centre where a CT scan and blood work would be available. The first specialist I spoke with, a neurologist, said, "I'd love to help you out, but I don't have a single bed here. Sorry." Click.

Next hospital. "Sorry, I don't have a bed." And the third and the fourth were the same. The fifth specialist was a gruff neurosurgeon. "Yeah, hi, so tell me the story exactly."

"Well, I have a fifty-year-old woman, diabetic, unconscious with stable vitals, query stroke, heart attack, intracranial bleed, I don't know to be honest."

"Well, tell me the workup that you have so far," she exuded impatience, implying that I had delivered a poorly told synopsis.

"I'm in a nursing station where the blood work has to be flown out—there is nothing in terms of a workup. Her ECG is normal." I felt as alone as the patient might have felt, lying unconscious and unaware of the family gathering around her.

Silence. Disbelief.

"Okay, fine. But just be aware that if this is a big, bad, intracranial bleed, then I'm not going to do anything as her prognosis would be poor and all I would be doing is prolonging her suffering, which I refuse to do. So if the family is prepared for this possibility, which it sounds like is very plausible, then that's fine. They need to understand she will possibly die alone in a foreign town rather than with her loved ones at her side."

"Understood. I'll talk to them and see what they say."

I put the phone on hold and attempted to walk convincingly on jellied legs back to the gathered family.

We were hoping the family would understand and come to terms with the imminent passing of their loved one. To spare them the harrowing journey of options that modern medicine allows. Choices that in many cases prolong someone's living misery and only postpone the inevitable, often by no more than a few hours or days. The postponement sometimes lasts much longer, however, with increased physical trauma to the body, and psychological trauma for the patient, family members, as well as medical staff.

With these thoughts circulating in my mind, talking to the family began anew. At this stage, a chorus of over forty people awaited my verbal conduction. Anxiety had bumped up another octave as I was about to have an end of life discussion for the first time since qualifying.

"So," I began, "at the present time I don't have a clear idea of what is going on with your [grand] mother; given that she has had really bad diabetes and her sugars have been quite high, she could have had a stroke, a bleed in the brain. The main thing we need in addition to blood work is imaging of the brain. There is a good chance that it may not be operable and she may be a long way away from you all, her loved ones, while we try and organize these tests down south. If you decide to send her, there is a very real chance that she will die alone with only one family member by her side and without your immediate love and affection. Now there is a small chance that everything will go well and she might recover, but the chances of that are pretty low right now. So what are your thoughts?" The decision was in the audience's hands now.

Silence. Disbelief.

They looked at me as if the grim reaper had just spoken to them. I was still warm, my palms were sweaty, my heart—palpable in my chest. I desperately tried to quickly assess their faces, their thoughts. I doubt they even heard half of what I said, let alone understood the half they did hear.

"Well?"

"So, Doc, do you think she'll live?"

Clearly, my explanation and intentions did not achieve the intended result. I tried again.

"Well, all I can say is, if this was my mother, I would make peace with her and be beside her here at home, rather than somewhere else alone. Take some time to decide what you want to do, but we may not have a lot of time. Also, remember that if someone's heart stops for any reason, CPR resuscitates less than 2 per cent of young, healthy people; now, older people who are not fit fare much worse than the young healthy ones, and if they survive, it will be with significant brain damage. Now, if her heart stops for any reason, which is a high chance, she will likely not survive. So having said this, do you want her to be full code (meaning all resuscitation interventions will be performed) if her heart stops for any reason?"

The answer was a resounding "Yes!" from one or two family members, followed by a room full of supportive nods. My gut reaction was sheer exasperation. I felt like I had spent the last twenty minutes peeing against the wind. I was fearful that I would be complicit in the physical assault of this poor woman in her last moments should she code in the next few minutes. On the other hand, it was an unpleasant feeling to be the bearer of bad news, but this was what all those years of training were hopefully preparing me for…?

So without a moment to waste, I returned back to the nursing station and was back on the phone arranging for the transfer to the neurosurgeon approximately four hours away by plane.

"Hello, yes, this is Dr. Mehta. When should there be a plane available next?"

"Less than an hour."

"Good, here is the name of the surgeon I'm sending this patient to. Greatly appreciated."

And so began the wait that terrifies new physicians when they first realize they are powerless and that a situation can deteriorate at any minute. To manage that anxiety and to prevent myself from pacing, I found documenting the events a productive distraction.

And so I furiously documented, illegibly but therapeutically, until the air paramedics arrived.

"Dr. Mehta, the paramedics are here."

"Great!" I replied, elated yet deflated.

They marched in, wheeling a stretcher and assessing my patient. I gave them the summary and made sure they knew where she was going.

"She's going where? Ah, crap! We may not have enough fuel to get there; we've been out flying all day."

"Whaddya mean you may not have enough fuel?" I asked in terror.

"Don't worry, Dr. Mehta—I'm sure there's a little extra from the boats around here. We'll manage."

The senior paramedic was jolly. Though I chuckled a little, I really didn't want to know how they fuelled the plane at this point—I just wanted them to take this woman off my hands and my mind. After they wheeled her onto the plane and made a few phone calls, the plane took off, much to my relief, and I went back to doing some charting.

*We'll manage. We'll manage.*

I guess we do.

# Dr. Aamir Bharmal

*Aamir Bharmal is a family physician with interests in improving health quality, decreasing rural-urban health disparities, and First Nations health. He practised full-scope, rural family medicine in Moose Factory and its five satellite communities along the west coast of James Bay, Ontario, from 2013 to 2014. He completed his undergraduate training in biology and medical sociology at the University of Calgary and medical school at the University of Alberta. Aamir is currently pursuing additional training in public health through the master of public health program at Johns Hopkins University and the public health and preventive medicine residency program at the University of Toronto.*

## Bingo

The pickup truck veered out of the way as she ran past the vehicle's grille. Having narrowly avoided collision, she turned her head and met the gaze of the driver whose expression was filled with annoyance and consternation. She barked twice at the truck as it blew up a plume of dust and drove up to the emergency department entrance.

Everyone had an opinion about her. Independent and territorial, all opinions, no matter how differing, agreed she was the alpha female of the island. In a show of both challenge and submission, her passing by was inevitably met with the barks of other dogs. To the stranger's eye, she appeared threatening and unpredictable, yet one would quickly realize that Bingo was just a protective, affectionate, stray dog.

Bingo stirred the hearts of the doctors and nurses on Moose Factory Island. A physician colleague of mine had taken her under his wing. She would come in for meals but stirred when kept inside too long. Bingo preferred to roam around the island and patrol the outdoors.

My running route trailed from the hospital to the garbage dump on the northern tip of the island. Despite being born and raised in Canada, rarely had I ever felt so surrounded by the trappings of Canadiana as on those runs. The run was a living illustration of the island's history. One of the country's oldest English-speaking settlements, Moose Factory's past was distinguished by the fur trade, the James Bay Cree, and its frontier location. Smells of cedar and cool northern breezes mixed with wheel-spun dust and potholes. Along the way lay cemeteries of the new- and long-dead, an abandoned church, and the nineteenth-century Hudson's Bay Staff House that juxtaposed the Quikstop gas station.

Bingo found me on my second day. I reacted with trepidation when she followed me on my run. I stopped running. She looked and then leapt towards me. I froze. She pawed against my legs and waited for my reaction. My petting her quickly defused the situation and allayed my concern.

As I resumed my previous pace, Bingo ran alongside. Making small detours from the path and into the thicket, she radiated energy. My runs were encouraged by her vitality.

Just south of the mouth of James Bay, Moose Factory's remote location raised significant challenges. On an island in the middle of the Moose River, the community was a ten-minute boat ride from the mainland. The hospital, Ontario's most remote, was originally built as a sanatorium. Little of the hospital's utilitarian exterior appearance had changed over the years. Situated on the south side of the island, the hospital served as the hub of medical care for six communities on the western coast of James Bay. Getting sick patients from these communities onto the island and medically unstable patients off the island was a challenge, further compounded by unpredictable and inclement weather conditions.

My first days of practice in Moose Factory were exciting but tumultuous. Even though I'd spent two months in the community as a medical resident and knew about the challenges of providing medical care there, it didn't make the experience any less daunting. I was fresh out of residency and on my first job as an independent family doctor. I wore many hats as a family physician in Moose Factory: delivering babies, working in the emergency department, managing in-patients on the floor, and working out of satellite community nursing stations in fly-in communities. I was attracted by the opportunity to continue to practise in all of the facets of family medicine I had trained in during my residency.

Despite the constantly shifting nature of my work—the possibility that a patient would suddenly become medically unstable, that the emergency helicopter could not fly, or an important piece of medical equipment was not working—Bingo was a constant. At the end of a long shift in the emergency room, she would find me on my walk home. Despite my unpredictable schedule and variable shift times over the week, Bingo intuitively knew when I was leaving the hospital. She would obediently wait on my porch as I entered my home, conspicuously waiting for a bowl of dog food to be doled out to her. Within moments of the bowl being set down, the contents were quickly devoured.

My 1.5-kilometre walk down Centre Road to the "Complex" where the island grocery store, post office, and administrative offices were housed started and ended with Bingo following closely behind. As we passed by houses along the way, other neighbourhood dogs stirred in their front yards. Small dogs followed her lead and discreetly followed from a distance. Larger dogs would cautiously bark at Bingo, shying away as she approached closer. I filled my grocery bags at the store with a week's wares while she waited at the exit of the Complex to accompany me on the way home.

In health, we are protected. It's a constant that we don't give any further thought to. Our bodies are the means to accomplishing tasks. We expect health to keep up with us, just as I expected Bingo to be waiting outside the hospital after my shift in the emergency department or when I stepped outside the grocery store with full grocery bags. Whether on a run or the twelfth hour of a hospital shift, our health is a silent given.

Fall transitioned to winter and the days got shorter and cooler. My colleague who gave Bingo shelter at night had to leave the community unexpectedly and indefinitely due to a family emergency. Bingo spent the next few weeks roaming the area around the hospital, intermittently barking and chasing after cars.

Bingo's overzealous nature caught up with her. The hospital maintenance manager sent out an email to all staff, indicating that there were multiple complaints about a dog running amok on hospital property and in the surrounding residential area. Bingo had been noted to act threateningly towards a child who was waiting outside for a school bus. "The black dog's owner" was asked to make sure that Bingo was supervised and restrained, and arrangements were to be made for the dogcatcher if the owner did not comply.

The physicians made arrangements for Bingo to be adopted and taken care of by a former physician working in southern

Ontario. A lab technician would be driving there in two weeks, and for the time being, Bingo would be tied up to the technician's porch so the dogcatcher wouldn't take her away. We were proud of finding a solution for Bingo, and were excited by the prospect that she would have the opportunity to run freely on a ranch in southern Ontario soon.

With the departure of a close colleague and Bingo's pending move, I realized how isolated Moose Factory really was. It was so unpredictable; the delicate health of sick patients, equipment failures, and general clinical volatility often made me feel powerless. So many factors of clinical practice were fleeting and out of my control. Carefully planned and coordinated out-of-town medical appointments could easily fall apart with inclement weather.

For patients in Moose Factory, taking care of their health was a significant undertaking. Attendance at out-of-town investigations and appointments was a major investment of time and energy. These appointments took them away from their family, their work, and sometimes their community. Flying to Kingston, Ontario, for a specialist visit was a whirlwind experience where a patient would be shuttled into a hospital and dropped into an unfamiliar culture. They may be barraged with a number of questions from health care providers for specific details they had given little previous thought to. Physician recommendations at the appointment could be incomprehensible. At times, patients returned to Moose Factory with little recollection of what had happened at these medical appointments, let alone why.

I'll never forget the last time I saw Bingo. Chained to a porch and about to be driven "down south," she let out whinnies and yelps as I approached from a distance. She attempted to run up to me but was held back by the chain around her neck.

Seeing Bingo constrained and powerless made me realize how fast things could change and how unpredictable life was. Mere weeks ago, Bingo had shelter and the freedom to roam around the island as she pleased. In the same way, my work had shown me how rapidly things changed for my patients. Disease had a way of quickly changing the constant and unnoticed to something all-encompassing, even finite.

Health can be fragile. Bingo demonstrated this. My colleague was a vital component to keeping a semblance of control over a "stray dog." When that constancy was lost, Bingo was given full rein and her behaviour came under the notice of community members. Suddenly, the black dog in the community who barked at cars and affectionately ran up to residents became a stray dog needing constraint.

Kneeling beside Bingo, I ruffled her fur. Her yelps subsided and she settled down. I sat in the snow beside her and took in the sounds of her breathing.

During sickness, health becomes a treasured memory. We're unsure of how much our physical and mental well-being affects us until it starts to show signs of wear. Patients have vividly recounted to me what they were able to do when they were healthy; their bodies work to bring them back to the paragon of health.

I imagine her at the ranch now. She's navigating through tall grasses and exploring surrounding fields. No longer barking after cars and avoiding possible collision, this island in the Moose River is but a distant memory.

**ONTARIO**

# Dr. Geordie Fallis

*Geordie Fallis began his education at Armour Heights Public School in Toronto in 1955. At the age of ten, he was elected president of the Red Cross for his Grade 5 class. Since then, it's been pretty much down-hill. He graduated from McMaster Medical School in 1975 and has enjoyed practising family medicine in many remote and not-so-remote settings. Currently, he's a staff physician with the Southeast Toronto Family Health Team, a staff physician at the Toronto East General Hospital in complex continuing care, and an assistant professor in family medicine at the University of Toronto. Some of "Veterinary Tales" was previously published in* From Testicles to Timbuktu: Notes from a Family Doctor *(Flawlis Publishing, 2013).*

## Veterinary Tales

My first job as a family doctor was in a small fishing village called Bella Coola in the Coast Mountains of British Columbia. We were the only medical show in town. The old hospital had twenty beds and serviced not only both the village and the local First Nation reserve but also some one thousand inhabitants up the valley to where the mountains began.

Once a week we would drive up the mountains to a smaller reserve called Anahim Lake. We would assist at a clinic run by a courageous nursing sister from Quebec, Sister Suzanne. When Sister Suzanne was in trouble, she would call us in Bella Coola. We called it "pamper time," because if she could not handle it, it was something bad, as she could handle most things!

The nearest secondary care hospital was hundreds of kilometres away in the ranching town of Williams Lake. Often times, we would send patients to the doctors there for more definitive treatment, but we could handle such things as dilation and curettage, appendectomies, and Caesarean sections. The nearest veterinarian was also located in Williams Lake. The latter situation posed some logistical problems for the inhabitants of the Bella Coola valley. Either they fixed the animal problems themselves or travelled to Williams Lake to visit the vet. If all else failed, they would contact us.

### Hung like a Horse

One evening when I was on call, one of the men from the reserve called and asked if I might help him out. He couldn't come to the hospital because it had to do with his horse. Apparently, the horse had tried to jump over a barbed wire fence. Unfortunately, he had caught his scrotum on the way down, resulting in a twenty-centimetre laceration on the horse's scrotal sac. There was no way I was going to attempt to sew the cut, unless the horse was totally immobilized. I had visions of being kicked in the head and rendered unconscious, or perhaps worse, dead.

Fortunately, the local pharmacist, Grant Edwards, had developed a keen interest in the pharmacology and treatment of animals. He had taken this on himself, knowing that the nearest vet was so far away. Grant had become very knowledgeable in the administration of a horse tranquillizer, Rompun (Xylazine), and felt fearless about its administration no matter the size of the animal. But the horse with the lacerated scrotum was his first patient. He assured me that he knew the right amount of anesthetic or amnesic agent that needed to be given.

He proceeded to give the medication through a very large vein on the horse's front leg. Within minutes, the horse was snoring and still standing. Not knowing how much time I had, I rolled onto my back like a car mechanic and lay under the animal. I put in the quickest running suture I had done in my fledgling medical career. The horse did not move. Two weeks later, we were told that the horse was doing well.

### Cat with a Prolapsed Uterus

One day, I got a call from the local owner of the dry goods store in Bella Coola. Her cat had delivered a litter of three and had a prolapsed uterus. This means that the womb had fallen out of the birth passage along with the last kitten. The woman had called the vet in Williams Lake and asked if she should drive the cat in to have it checked out. The vet said he did not think there was a need to drive the difficult road in winter if the local doctor would be willing to resolve the problem. All that was required, according to the vet, was to push the uterus back up into the vagina and put in a purse-string suture. A purse-string suture is a continuous running suture that pinches off a hole or orifice, in this case the vagina. Hence, the call I received from the local proprietor. She told me what the vet had said, and I said I would be more than willing to help out, as long as the pharmacist would put the cat to sleep.

After his success with the horse, Grant had no hesitation in putting the cat to sleep. After the cat was well anesthetized, I was able to push the uterus back into the birth canal and do a purse-string stitch. The woman was very thankful that I was able to do this, and the cat seemed no worse for wear.

Unfortunately, Grant had given the cat a very hefty dose of the tranquilizer. It did not wake up for two full days. When it did, the woman said that the cat appeared to be bearing down as if she was still in labour. I reassured her that the uterus was quite empty when I put things back into place and went off hiking.

But the cat continued to bear down as if she were pushing in the third stage of labour. The owner decided that she had to do something and cut the purse-string suture. Out came the fourth kitten of the litter in very good shape. Unfortunately, the cat prolapsed again. This time, when the woman brought the cat to the clinic, it was quite obvious that the cat had a bicornate uterus. Not realizing that cats have two horns to the uterus, this meant that when I pushed the uterus back up inside and sewed things off, I had no idea there was another kitten in there. Fortunately, the kitten survived and developed normally. The cat also did well with its second surgery.

News travels very quickly up the Bella Coola valley. In no time my obstetrical practice tailed off precipitously. Word got out that it was not a great idea to go and see the new young doctor at the hospital. He sews up vaginas when there are babies still inside.

**ONTARIO**

# Dr. James Yan

*James Yan was born in Vancouver, British Columbia, where he com-*
*pleted his undergraduate degree in honours physiology with a minor*
*in commerce. He graduated medical school from the Schulich School*
*of Medicine at Western University. In addition to his studies, he was*
*very engaged in student leadership, volunteering for his class council*
*and serving as an executive officer for the Ontario Medical Students*
*Association Council. After medical school, he began training in ortho-*
*pedic surgery at McMaster University. He plans to train towards*
*working in a rural community centre to improve access to surgical*
*care. Outside of medicine, James greatly enjoys the outdoors and activ-*
*ities such as snowboarding, hiking, biking, skiing, and photography.*

## The Student

The train rolls into town around midnight. The first thing the
student notices is how dark the night is. The ambient fluorescent
glow that lights and similarly mutes the night sky in the city
is missing. Walking out of the carriage, the humidity hits him
first, gluing his shirt to his back. The heat comes next. It's like
walking into a greenhouse. The shirt quickly becomes drenched.

He meets a classmate who had agreed to pick him up from the station.

"Already feels different from back home."

"The heat? Yeah, I noticed that, too, last night when I got in."

They drive off to find the house the student will be staying at for the month. This takes a while, as the low amount of street lighting makes the address difficult to spot, despite the house's proximity to the hospital.

The new arrival is surprised when they finally find the house. In his mind's eye he had imagined some sort of lofty hotel, a posh inn, or a bed and breakfast. Instead, he is met with an old, refurbished, residential house. It has the essentials but not much more—the room has only a bed and an ancient armoire, and a small lamp in the corner for light. These are not the accommodations the student had expected. But it's late, and the travel and heat have exhausted him. He simply changes his clothes, finds some clean sheets, and collapses onto the bed.

• • •

The town stands transformed in the light of morning. The hospital is on the other bank of the river. The student can see it from the house. It's a short walk. Nonetheless, the humidity, it lingers. Accusingly, his eyes fall on the winding viridian strip of river as he walks across the bridge, looking to blame any source of moisture for the muggy weather. He contemplates jogging the rest of the way to shorten his time out in the heat, but decides that the extra energy expenditure would be worse. The air-conditioned hospital is a welcoming oasis.

Fortunately, he is early and can cool off before the orientation meeting for the visiting trainees. Unfortunately, only the orientation is at the hospital that day and it is another long trek to where the pediatrics clinic is. In a town where infrastructure was planned around automotive travel, commuting by foot is time-consuming. Despite the heat, the student hurries this time—it is close to the time when the clinic opens. Rule One of clerkship—it was drilled into his head—*never be late*.

"The Daily Planet" reads the sign outside. The clinic is in the basement of an old newspaper building. *Well, here goes.* If nothing else, maybe he'll meet Superman.

He walks downstairs.

The clinic is busy. Four pediatricians share the practice. The student rotates a day with each of them during the week, usually the one who is holding the pager for any consults that come from the hospital. Once a week, a special chronic disease management day occurs—looking at diabetes and asthma, for example. There is always something for the clerk to do—a week in and he is starting to feel accustomed to it.

It is now lunchtime and the student is catching up on dictations between bites of a wrap: "…please end dictation." His thumb slides the "off" button on the silver Dictaphone assigned to him. No fancy transcription service here. The audio notes will be typed out later. The morning cases are done. He has a few minutes to himself before the afternoon begins.

It's a nice day for a walk—the sun is out and the river is a swollen vein of emerald surging with new runoff. The student strolls down to a local deli near the clinic. He grabs a coffee and has a quick chat with the owner, Dave, before heading back. It is warm, and the humidity has dissipated with the recent rainfall.

Morning rounds with patients, dictations, lunch, afternoon patients, dictations. Home. He has the routine figured out. It's busy, but he's getting used to it.

• • •

Today, he and a colleague sit with a mother and her son. The boy's condition is not life-threatening, but the news is life-changing. The mother's attempts to be stoic are betrayed by her trembling eyes. The pediatrician is trying to explain what the diagnosis means, but the mother hears only one word.

Autism.

Words slip by. The mother retreats, withdraws into herself. The student imagines the worries and anxiety building up in her mind: travel distances, costs and expenses, taking time off work. His mouth opens tentatively, but no sounds come out. His gaze turns away to the wall. He feels embarrassed that he has nothing to offer.

His colleague, however, takes pause. Her eyes glimmer knowingly. The silence draws the mother out of her mental maelstrom. Attention refocused, the pediatrician goes over again with the mother a new plan and the options available to her. She smiles, "It'll be okay." The mother's eyes turn towards her boy—he's been playing with a truck the whole time. She nods. She's starting to believe it will be, too.

• • •

Late afternoons are for summer storms. Wind whips branches against windows, howling past buildings. Old glass panes shake, and wood frames warp under the strain. A sharp staccato of rain bullets bombard the roofs. Lightning and thunder blind and deafen.

While a tempest plays on outside, the student stretches out peacefully on worn hardwood panels. He's found a small yoga studio, which appeals to his urban sensibilities. Flowing into another pose, he times his breathing with the gusts heard overhead.

Flickering lights above and the scent of sweat and pine surround him as he relaxes into a lotus. *Rural medicine is kind of like this moment right now*, he muses. The rest of clerkship can be thrashing out there, a big commotion trying to beat down everything in its path—but here you can find your centre.

You have the space to breathe.

There is wellness here.

• • •

Four weeks. It has passed so quickly. His bags packed, it's time for the student to lock up the house one last time. He is greeted once again by the heat. A mild hum of cicada drones on in the background. A few beads of sweat are already forming.

His classmate is waiting outside. They load up their bags and drive off. Over the narrow bridge that has become so familiar. Out, fast, onto the dusty roads headed home. It's a long drive back. The town has already disappeared behind fields of corn in the rear-view mirror. The car hits the highway and his classmate turns to him.

"So what did you think? Ready to be back in the big city?"

"Hah, you know what?" the student responds. "It was a good time. Never experienced that before. We don't see medicine in this setting all that much."

"True. Do you think you'll be back anytime soon?"

"Well, who knows? I would like to try some fishing out of the river," he chuckles.

*Who* really *knows,* he thinks to himself...*I've crossed enough bridges over this past month. I'll get to that one eventually.*

**ONTARIO**

# Dr. Dan Eickmeier

*Dan Eickmeier was born and raised in rural southern Ontario. He learned that he knew everything at McMaster University and the University of Western Ontario, where he completed his family medicine residency. A realization of his naivety began in Kirkland Lake, Ontario, in 2004, and he became fully aware of it in Seaforth, Ontario, in 2007. His wife, Laura, and daughter, Freya, keep his ego in line. Away from medicine, he distracts himself with skiing, bicycling, cooking, and listening to music on vinyl records.*

## I Figured It Would Be Easy

When I first agreed to write something for this collection, I figured it would be easy. I rant about rural medicine all the time. How hard could it be to come up with a couple thousand words to encapsulate my experience over the past ten years in rural medicine? Then the first deadline came and went, then the second. Maybe this wouldn't be quite so easy.

I like to do stuff. I like to figure stuff out.

My dad was a general contractor and my mother a small-town Grade 1 teacher. In their respective jobs, they just figured out what needed to be done and did it. My dad could build, plumb, wire, and design a house. My mom figured out the parts of the curriculum that mattered and just helped her students learn. Sure, my parents would get help when they had to, due to time or, occasionally, complexity, but they could get the basics done on their own.

I guess that is what made me the doc I am today. I see it as almost a failure when I have to send a patient to the specialist. I am always thinking, "What else could we try?" I don't know if this is better than other ways of practising, but it is the only way I really know how to do things. Fortunately, working in rural medicine meshes quite nicely with that attitude. Unfortunately, I think this way of practising is rapidly fading into the sunset. Hospitalists, ER specialists, office family docs, nursing home docs, walk-in docs, etc., etc.—I am not sure what the future holds for "young dinosaurs" like us. I hope there will always be a place for us, but I don't know what it will be. Is there a way to live a balanced life without narrowing your practice? If not, the young dinosaurs will face an early extinction.

I am not really sure if I am a young physician anymore. In a few months I will have been in practice for ten years. I still think of myself as young, but the twenty-four-hour ER shifts and being on call for twenty-four hours every four days is starting to take its toll on my body and my soul. Now I'm a mentor for the "new guys," but who is mentoring me to be a mentor? Avoiding the administrative jobs has become impossible. Can I even remember the halcyon days of the first couple of years of practice? I'm not sure. All I can really say is that I'm still at it, and I am still a reasonably full-scope, rural generalist and I can't really imagine being anything else.

Growing up in a small town in Ontario's agricultural heartland, I had wanted to be a doctor since I was twelve years old, and the only kind of doctor I ever knew was an "old school" small-town generalist. Obstetrics, emergency medicine, anesthesia, in-patient work, nursing homes, the docs of my childhood did it all.

Throughout high school and university, I focused on doing what I needed to do to get into med school. After a couple of bumps in the road, I made it. Through med school I did everything as "rurally" as I could. I was a bit of an oddball in a Hawaiian shirt, but it never seemed to matter when I was out in the country. When I finally finished my residency and it was time to "choose my grown-up life," my wife and I decided to take a leap and go outside our comfort zone. We relocated to northern Ontario and spent three interesting years in Kirkland Lake. There were many wonderful things about our life there, but there were also challenges that turned out to be too great to make it long-term. Back to the agricultural heartland for us, and that's where we've been for the past seven years. We added a daughter. We renovated an old church into a home. We lost people. We gained friends.

As I sit here, I am trying to figure out what it means to me to be a small-town doc. Is it the police showing up on my doorstep in the middle of the night because the hospital couldn't get through and they needed my help? Is it the patients that ask about their results in the grocery store or while I'm mowing the lawn? Is it the tolerance of my Hawaiian shirts, long hair, and bushy beard? Is it knowing that the only way to really be "off call" is to be a long way from everything? Or maybe it's the coffee and sandwiches that the local restaurant owner dropped off at the hospital after I looked after him in the ER? How about watching a CME (continuing medical education) video on YouTube for a procedure I haven't done in years, then confidently walking into the room and just doing it as if I've done it a thousand times because it was what needed to be done? Maybe it's the colleagues (even if they are virtual ones) who provided solace when a patient who I thought I had a connection with after saving his life crushed my spirit by complaining to the administration about a hole in my favourite old cardigan. How about the gift from an unemployed paraplegic patient for treating his incontinence and other "GU" (genitourinary) issues with dignity? Or maybe a certain, particularly memorable in-patient who had pneumonia, whose room I went into to see how he was coming along. I had asked him, "Are you back to normal?" (He had been hallucinating during the worst of it.) He said, "What the hell is normal? It is just a perception of reality. Your normal and my normal will never be the same." I rephrased the question: "Are you back to your normal?" To which he responded, "Sure as shit I am and ready to get out of here, and, by the way, you are the closest to normal that I have yet found amongst doctors." I am pretty sure that was a compliment. That's how I took it anyway.

• • •

Now the challenging question: Do I love my work? I'm not really sure if I do or not. Elements of it I definitely love: the rush of the ER; the excitement of learning something new or researching a particularly challenging patient's condition; connecting with a patient in the office when they have their epiphany that only they can really change their health for the better; having a crusty old patient give me a teddy bear to take home to my daughter for her birthday; having a patient ask to give me a hug for all the care I provided for her husband on her first office visit after his death.

Then there are the parts I hate: medical politics; guide-line-based practice; the use of evidence-based medicine to ask the wrong questions; the nights away from home; the missed events with family; the expectations of what a physician should look and sound like.

So what is the balance? I can't say I always love what I do, and I have even looked at a lot of other options and have come pretty darn close to making a switch. But even with all those other potentially attractive options, I am still working away as a small-town general practitioner. I am not sure I've found a satisfying balance—that is the honest truth—but what I have is really the best I can hope for.

**MANITOBA**

# Dr. Aleem Jamal

*Like others in the 1970s, Aleem Jamal's parents were expelled from Uganda under the dictatorship of Idi Amin, and came to Canada as refugees. They settled in a quiet and small community, the village of Brechin, Ontario, where both Aleem and his sister were raised. As Ismaili Muslims, they were brought up with the values of generosity, brotherhood, and compassion, and a strong emphasis was placed on education. Aleem pursued post-secondary education in Kingston, Ontario, where he completed a bachelor of science at Queen's University. Continuing his education "across the pond," he completed medical training at the Royal College of Surgeons in Ireland. After graduation, he moved back to Canada to complete family medicine training in the Northern Remote stream at the University of Manitoba. Outside of his academic pursuits, he enjoys the great outdoors, travelling, and experiencing different cultures and environments.*

## No More Training Wheels

The following is the account of my first call as an attending physician. The story is more about the doctoring than about the medicine. As I have quickly learned, medicine does not change from place to place. Rather, growth as a physician occurs amid the context in which you practise.

I was excited to return to work in a place where I spent time as a resident, in the beautiful community of Norway House, Manitoba. Norway House, one of the original Hudson's Bay Company trading posts, is a rural community with a population of around eight thousand to nine thousand people. It is located about 450 kilometres north of Winnipeg on the eastern bank of Nelson River. It shares its name with Norway House Cree Nation (Kinosao Sipi Cree Nation), and has both a chief and a mayor.

Working in northern Manitoba comes with its own interesting set of challenges, and it is not always a comfortable place to be. Harnessing the emotional stress that comes with working in an under-resourced and isolated area while managing the unpredictable nature of any given workday can be a deterrent to many. But that's what I found appealing. After taking four months off after graduating, I started to work in the same rural environment where I had done my mandatory rotation as a resident. Like others before me, I returned to a community that I truly adored while providing a service in a part of Canada that desperately needed physicians.

My first few days back at the northern clinic were smooth. I saw many of the typical everyday conditions seen in any urban centre: coughs, colds, sore throats, diabetes, hypertension. I can still vividly remember the brisk November morning walking into the ER for my first day on call. I was excited but nervous, a little consumed with trepidation of the unknown. Funnily enough, as I pondered the plethora of emergencies I might potentially encounter, I was not the least bit worried about the numerous wolf sightings near the hospital, which concerned the locals so much they were keeping their children and dogs indoors. I don't know why they didn't frighten me; I like to think it was because doctors tend to focus on other people's welfare more than their own, but it was more likely that the fear of what I had to potentially deal with trumped any fear of actual physical harm.

Thankfully, my first day on call was quite banal in the beginning, and many of the early cases I saw were of the "urgent care" type rather than a true emergency. For a brief moment I resolved to believe that my first stint in the ER would not be so bad.

Then walked in Mrs. Anderson, a splendid woman, polite and humorous, who I had the pleasure to meet and treat. Mrs. Anderson had come into the emergency room short of breath, with an oxygen saturation in the nineties. She was also tachycardic but with a stable blood pressure. She was a known asthmatic, but after listening to her chest and not hearing any sounds, and percussing stony dull notes on her right side, I sent her off for imaging. The X-ray confirmed my suspicions and revealed a fluffy white-coloured right lung— in other words, a massive, right-sided, pleural effusion. I knew her chest needed a tube put into it immediately to save her life. I had seen a couple chest tube insertions during residency but only assisted with one, well over a year earlier.

Luckily, I had a lot of backup in the clinic that afternoon. One family medicine resident on rotation was a former cardiothoracic surgery resident who was experienced with tube thoracostomies. He walked me through the procedure, ensuring that I did not miss any important steps. Considering this was my first call, this alone would have gone down in my books as a great return to rural medical practice. However, midway through the chest tube insertion, an unstable patient came in with acute onset of chest pain, hypotension, and tachycardia. Just my luck, I thought to myself. As I was stabilizing one patient, literally having both hands tied, another one who needed immediate attention came into the ER. When it rains, it pours.

Again, by luck—or if you're a person of faith, divine intervention—the chief of staff just happened to be wandering around. He had overheard the buzz of an unstable patient, saw that I was in the middle of a chest tube insertion, and, without hesitation or call for assistance, came in to start managing the patient with the acute chest pain. I felt my pulse slow and the throbbing in my head begin to dissipate. Once I had finished handling the tube thoracostomy, sent off the pleural fluid for analysis, and quickly wrote down admission orders, I headed over to the other unstable patient, who was now in the hands of my colleague.

Mr. Brennan was a pleasant forty-year-old gentleman, with many family and friends in the community. He had recently been diagnosed with biventricular heart failure, with a left ventricular ejection fraction of less than 35 per cent, poor. He was taking anticoagulants for a clot found in his heart, and was scheduled for follow-up for either an implantable cardioverter-defibrillator or cardiac resynchronization therapy. Upon arrival to the emergency room, as stated above, he was tachycardic and had an unreadable blood pressure with the automated blood pressure cuff. The nurses had a difficult time getting a peripheral line in, as his vasculature was completely constricted, but they eventually managed. Our initial attempts to volume resuscitate with IV fluids were unsuccessful; we needed vasopressor (a medication to raise blood pressure) support. That day, my first day on call, my chief of staff gave me the quintessential "head nod"—a tacit acknowledgement of implied trust and a confirmation for me to proceed with putting in a central venous catheter. Then, without a second glance, the chief of staff went on to call Lifeflight (the air ambulance, with a group of obstetricians, critical care staff, and emergency physicians providing twenty-four-hour care) to help get Mr. Brennan to a tertiary care centre for further management.

Using ultrasound, and with the help of my trusted former cardiothoracic resident, I attempted to put in a central internal jugular (IJ) line. This would only be my second ultrasound-guided IJ line; my first would have been almost a year before. I initially had the correct placement, but just as I was about to thread the guidewire, the patient became agitated and coughed and I missed the placement of the wire. At this point I decided it was best to aim for peripheral access in order to salvage the central access until the Lifeflight physician arrived. We achieved a palpable pulse of 55 mmHg using peripheral vasopressors, which was markedly improved from his previously absent systolic pressure. I thanked both the chief of staff and the resident and urged them to go back to their posts. Collectively, we had done everything we could to keep the patient alive and stable until Lifeflight arrived.

When Lifeflight did arrive, the ICU physician also encountered difficulty acquiring a central line, which provided me with a bit of comfort over my failed attempt; at least I could see this wasn't an easy task, even for the most experienced of doctors. Eventually, as we were intubating and getting access, the patient coded (entered cardiopulmonary arrest). My heart sank, knowing that few people come out unscathed at this point. My training in Ireland and Manitoba afforded a lot of different opportunities, but I had somehow made it through my medical training with only having observed a few codes—never had I run a code on my own patient.

Time seemed to speed up. After twenty minutes of continuous CPR, and the usual slate of medications, we finally achieved a palpable and self-sustaining pulse, but it went by in a flash. Although he was alive, I remember feeling uneasy about him surviving the flight to Winnipeg. The critical care doc and I went to speak with the family and provide an update: Mr. Brennan was in very critical condition and may not make the flight back.

He had a large, supportive family, all of whom were waiting in the ER. As news of his condition spread, the array of emotions threaded together to create a wall—I slammed into it hard when I entered the room to deliver the update. Their eyes were filled with desperation, their lips tightly puckered, and the room was pin-drop silent. You could see and feel each member of the family leaning in attentively. They were aching for positive news. Any shred of positive news would have alleviated their pain, but just as I began to speak, we all heard the shrill sound of a nurse screaming: *Code!*

I remember the scene very vividly: just as we were saying the words "may not survive the flight," the nurse's cry interrupted us. Without explanation, we rushed back into the emergency room, but not without seeing the fear and apprehension cross the bewildered faces of the family.

We were unable to keep him alive.

After another thirty minutes of resuscitation, we simply could not revive him. It was then that time passed slowly. I remember secretly hoping and praying that this gentle and kind man would somehow make it back to life. The harsh reality of the profession we are in is that things do not always turn out the way we want them to. One of the most difficult things I have had to do was to explain to the family that their cherished relative was here no more. It seemed as though the family's emotion and grief had penetrated the hearts of everyone in the hospital and community.

After the family had left, the death certificate was filled out and the body was sent to the morgue. The six hours left of my shift seemed to pass by unnoticed. There was a feeling of calmness and silence, as if the entire community knew what had happened and were paying their respects by keeping well. By the end of the day, I had experienced not only my first call but my first chest tube, my second central line, my first run code, and my first death. Death under my watch, under my care.

The next couple of call shifts seemed less intense, even though I had to run a code on another patient and fly back with a patient on a medevac because Lifeflight was busy on another call. My nerves were still a bit shaky, my voice still trembled, but I definitely felt more confidence in myself—not only because of my previous experiences but also because of the people and support around me.

I learned a lot that night, about myself and about being a physician in the North. In remote or rural areas you cannot help but become part of the communities you work in; the people you treat are an extension of yourself. You learn that you cannot expect to know everything all at once; you learn to be humble. Ego can be the Achilles heel of the medical profession and a potential block from transitioning good doctors into great ones. More than being a disadvantage to yourself, it can be a detriment to the patients you treat. It is important to ask for help, whether from a specialist, another colleague, a nurse, a resident, or even a med student—they all become part of your team, your support, and your lifeline. All doctors, no matter how great or experienced, are a work in progress. They call it *practising* medicine for a reason.

I cannot conclude this story without thanking all of the people who contribute to the growth and development we go through as physicians: the allied health care staff among the rural, remote, and urban centres who make our days rewarding and valuable; the wonderful education—both medical and nonmedical—we have been blessed to receive from the myriad teachers and mentors across the globe; and last, but not least, our family and friends. I don't think any physician could ever make it to where they are without all their love and continued support. We are blessed to be in a profession in which we will always be challenged and driven to learn more; patients will not always have textbook presentations and medicine is never truly mastered.

I hope that rural and northern medicine is always part of my career, no matter where I end up in life, and I thank everyone who led me—and all the other rural and remote health care professionals—down this road less travelled.

**MANITOBA**

# Dr. Sandra Wiebe

*Sandra Wiebe grew up on a farm in Mather, Manitoba, where her mother was a teacher and her father did various jobs and stayed home raising the family. It was only as an adult that she decided to become a doctor and she completed her medical training in Winnipeg, Manitoba, in 2009. Her postgraduate training was completed in Fort St. John, British Columbia. Concurrently with medical school, residency, and during her first few months of independent work she found time to give birth to her four children. Her husband is now a full-time parent, having given up his engineering career in order to commit full-time to their children. In August 2013, she moved to Neepawa, Manitoba, to begin her practice. In her spare time she loves to be outside and looks forward to gardening, camping, and biking. Outside of work, family, and leisure pursuits, her passion lies in environmentalism and faith.*

## The Best Years of My Life

Our home is thirty years old, a "lodge style" home with pine everywhere, surrounded by an oak-covered prairie creek bank. It is going to undergo a large renovation to suit our family of six, but other than its current interior layout, it suits us perfectly because it's close to town but has space for the big garden and the outdoor ventures that we dream about.

We have so much ahead of us.

As I sit down on a folding chair next to our fireplace, I begin to reflect. I'm trying to describe a day in my life as a new rural doctor in 2014. Two nights ago was my last call night and it comes to mind as eventful, as well as reasonably representative of my jumbled-up life.

I get home after midnight after seeing a child with a puffy sore eye. It was a peri-orbital cellulitis and the child and mother have since been transferred to Winnipeg where they can get a scan, specialist assessment, and surgery, if necessary. I had decided to give it a chance to settle with an intravenous anti-biotic overnight and if, by some stroke of luck, it settled over-night, spare them the transfer.

Afebrile, normal vitals, and it didn't look *too* swollen—really, what experience do I have with peri-orbital cellulitis? None. I remember two things from a lecture: 1) the condition is serious; and 2) the picture shown to illustrate it. The nonmedical factors I have a lot of personal familiarity with: concern about your child and navigating multiple demanding roles. I distinctly remem-ber that the mother's clothes were not very clean or matching. Neither are mine when I leave quickly at random times of day to go to the hospital.

The case before that was a gastrointestinal bleed to whom we gave our two units of emergency blood; the patient had improved a lot with the transfusion but unfortunately died from rebleed-ing the next day in the secondary hospital. I want to remember her husband and son because I am going to see them again—if nowhere else than in the community. He was a brown-haired man, dressed from work in coveralls that said "Shane's Shop"; he was appropriately nervous, and asked me straight out if she would die. Their blond son looked to be in his early twenties and said almost nothing.

It's two days later and my life is going on as usual.

I sometimes stop a minute and think about this. Someday it will be my turn to *not* just move on.

On my way home that night, I stop in at the clinic to treat my own plantar wart. I have been taking Tylenol and limping some mornings, so it's time to try to treat it, and I might as well do it at midnight, as my wind-down activity—I struggle to take the time during the day anyway. I'm glad that I already have a sense of comfort in "my" clinic building. I wonder what these feelings will include over the years—resentment? Pride? Dread? Love? Fatigue?

The next morning, I wake up in our large, upstairs, pine bedroom. Quiet, across the room, is our roommate, a twenty-month-old, whose crib is tucked behind a flimsy divider. My newly turned four-year-old son is nestled between my husband and me. I got lucky and had no calls overnight after the young boy with the sore eye.

I slip out and shower.

It's better if my husband and I are up before the children, but, really, it seldom happens. I skip the almost mandatory latte that my husband always makes for me. We both love our lattes; it's our little moment of pretending to sit and enjoy a warm, morning coffee. Sometimes I freeze-frame a morning view of our kitchen—my husband standing with a bunch of containers at the island, packing one to three lunches that are acceptable to our allergy-ridden school; two to three children opening drawers, pushing trucks, or laying on the floor while generating not-quite-endless cries, requests, questions, and general noise. It won't be long and I'll have a teenager view.

I do hospital rounds in the morning. Currently, I am one of six doctors in town and I'm secretly keen to get to know my colleagues. Two of us always round in the morning, three always during midday, and the other one, whenever he can fit it into his variously scheduled day. I have noticed since my arrival that this old hospital—almost ramshackle—was actually built to take advantage of the town's view over an eastward-looking ridge. That part is nice for patients, along with the proximity and familiarity. Sometimes old things can be attractive—this hospital is not one of those things. It looks piecemeal inside and out, and its age is apparent at a glance. That said, I am mostly indifferent to its inevitable replacement right now. My feelings about that will change when the time gets closer, but I also know they will not factor into decisions about it.

There is nothing very exciting about morning rounds, although I briefly round on the boy from last night and realize I have to properly address him later. There is a man who is from an even smaller community one hundred kilometres away. He had a stroke and we have a physiotherapist here five days a week instead of the once a week in his hometown. I "add" insulin to his chart, as I think it will help him, at which time he tells me he's been on insulin for decades. It wasn't on his incoming list of medications.

Two of my patients are elderly women who used to see the GP surgeon who worked here for three decades; he announced his retirement the week I arrived, and moved away within a month and a half. These are wonderful women, gracious to me. I struggle to accept the gratitude of the older one, well into her nineties, that I am willing to be her doctor. I don't do much for her other than pay attention to the details of her health and talk to her about it. She has a niece who has come to visit her and is highly independent despite multiple physical disabilities. I hope that as I get more confident and familiar with my patients and my practice I can more comfortably fulfill the role of "being there" for them. Demographically, I'm dissimilar to their prior GP, but I don't think that's of any significance for these women. As far as I know, they simply want a competent doctor there for them.

After my rounds, I go to the clinic. My patient list is only twelve or fourteen in number for the morning. It includes an eighty-something-year-old man in great health with questions about what I call "GERD" (gastroesophageal reflux disease), and a well, nine-month-old girl with a cough, who has just returned from the Philippines with her parents—so far this morning, my job is easy. I see another little baby of Filipino parents. I love to see them because she is growing and it reminds me that I was part of a truly life-saving event at her birth. After careful consultation locally, and alerting and training our hospital staff as to what to do if the mother arrived bleeding, we delivered this woman with a large posterior complete placenta previa in our own hospital. The baby was not really quite term, but I knew there was a reason for it, and now they are both doing well and the baby is growing and recovering from anemia.

The afternoon is "procedures" at the hospital. The first job is to transfer the boy. There is a hassle with how to get an ambulance. Everything from private vehicle to air ambulance is on the table at some point, and, eventually, it's settled on my first choice: our very competent ambulance land crew can take him.

I do relatively little by way of procedures, though my appetite grows as I continue to get better and learn more. This afternoon I am doing a Vandenbos, a removal of a chunk of skin around the nail. It goes well, and between stints of light-headedness, the young man is full of bravado. I know how to do this procedure almost exclusively because of YouTube, which I do not tell the patient or the medical student helping me. One of my colleagues in residency taught himself with that great YouTube video, and encouraged me to do the same; another made me do the procedure on her own sore toe. I did and now I can help someone with an otherwise annoying persistent problem. Maybe I'm not so different from the hardened generations past. You don't get taught many of the things you need to know; you figure it out with the means you have.

Because I only have the one procedure in the afternoon, I am home early at 4:00 p.m., as opposed to my usual 6:30, and

I get to play with the kids. My set includes an eight-year-old daughter and three sons, who are currently five, four, and one. I unpack my things and go upstairs to hug my daughter, sitting in the rocking chair with her new turquoise glasses on, reading a horse encyclopedia. After a few tussles with the boys, and talking to my husband about how discouraged he is by our expensive heating bill—it has been an exceptionally cold Manitoba winter—the younger two boys and I decide to go for a walk. I have forgotten my boots at the clinic, so after packing up the one-year-old and zipping up the four-year-old, I pack up in my mismatched snow pants and...runners—definitely not a warm, satisfactory way to go out into -30°C weather. I then drive to pick up my boots from the clinic, and fill up the van for my husband, who is driving the forty-five minutes to visit his parents tomorrow. We have a very short walk out to our "pasture" along the path through the snow. It follows the well-treed bank. Then we go in for the casserole that my husband cooked. We dream of getting animals, but we've not even been here for a year and we have a long way to go to get to that stage.

After the kids are in bed, I can go for another walk, this time in the dark on the hard-packed snow on our lane and then down the road. I settle myself again from my anxiety about a pregnant woman from the next town whose baby I was going to deliver but who developed hypertension, which I suspect will transition into pre-eclampsia (high blood pressure and protein in the urine) and require more urgent action. I've done the right investigations and don't need to transfer her—yet. As usual, I stew about my worst case: I watched someone hemorrhage to death for the first time following a high-speed highway collision. I often mentally recount details of what went wrong and all I learned from it.

Sometimes I think about how the messy house only bothers me when I'm below a certain busyness threshold. Then my thoughts turn to my personal unresolved dilemmas: How am I going to find a little space to be myself in this community? What will our children learn from us as we build our lives here? I'm not worried. I know I just need to proceed with respect and care.

I'm sure I slept well that night because I was, in fact, tired from the night before.

According to one of the surgeons I trained with, these are the best years of my life. The jury is still out as far as I'm concerned, especially as I sort through the inevitable petty politics of the job and transition out of the cycle of pregnancy and nursing into a (slightly) less interrupted life. But what he said is a good reminder to appreciate my luck: we were able to have the children that my husband and I wanted to; I have security as a doctor and the privilege to connect with so many different people; and I have fantastically interesting places to work and live. If my life stopped now, I couldn't complain. (Not that I wouldn't.)

# Dr. Lewis Draper

*Lewis Draper was born in Wallasey, Cheshire, across the Mersey from Liverpool in the United Kingdom. In Glasgow, where he attended university, he met his wife Erika, a Swiss Jewish woman and Holocaust survivor. He practised in Nigeria and Glasgow before moving to Saskatchewan. While in Saskatchewan, he practised in Wadena, Lafleche, and Gravelbourg. Lewis is the author of two books and does work as a locum family physician in Regina, Saskatchewan.*

## Monty

I could hear the screaming as I came in through the front door. The nurse was waiting for me at her station and followed me as I strolled into the X-ray room.

"Oh Doctor!" wailed the mother before I could say a word.

"He was in his walker in the kitchen and he fell with it down the basement stairs. Someone must have left the door open. I think he broke his leg. It's a funny shape and he won't let me touch it." She looked at me as if imploring me to say it wasn't so.

"Let's wait and see what the X-ray shows," I replied, "maybe it's not as bad as you think. Babies are a lot tougher than you think."

I comforted her as well as I could without committing myself to raise any false hopes but secretly thinking to myself it could as easily have been a broken neck, and then we would have been in trouble. The little fellow was eleven months old and I was not, as yet, as familiar with the family as I should have been, as the mother pointed out that I had delivered him.

There was a clink as the dark room door was unlocked and Clarice emerged with still wet X-rays clipped on their frames, trailing a stream of rinsing fluid across the room to the viewing box. One glance at her face and I knew the worst was true and began to brace myself for it.

"Well, let's see what we've got." I smiled as reassuringly as I could as I held the pungent films up to the light. "It seems to be a fracture of the shaft of the femur just below the hip joint." "Oh, sorry," I said to the parents as they crowded in for a better look. "Here just below the joint, see?" I pointed it out to them and showed them the difference on the other leg. Bad enough, but not catastrophic. The pelvis looked intact and the joint was not involved. "He'll be mended by the time his birthday comes around."

"Will he need an operation, Doctor?" asked his mother, fearfully.

"No, and he won't need a cast. He is going to be in hospital for about three weeks in traction and about a week after that he should be right as rain."

Louise the nurse gave me a quizzical, sidelong glance.

"Right then, I'll need a roll of three-inch Elastoplast strapping, a bottle of Friars' Balsam, a three-inch tensor bandage, and two wooden blocks about three inches square and an inch thick. Oh, and a drip stand."

"What do you want in the drip, Doctor? Normal saline?"

"No, nothing," I replied mysteriously. I was on solid ground here, having seen a similar fracture at Sick Kids Hospital in Glasgow. "If you can't find any wooden blocks, get hold of Edgar.

He'll find us some offcuts." Edgar was the local carpenter who did all the odd jobs for us at the hospital.

"Now while we are waiting for the nurse with the hardware, let's have a good look at the lad and make sure there's nothing else going on. He is a sturdy lad and looks all right, but we have to make sure there's nothing else damaged. His head is fine, the fontanelle is still just open and it is very elastic. Now otoscope, check his eardrums, and they are intact with no blood behind them. Can you hold his head, Daddy? He'll feel more secure in your hands. Pupils equal, regular, reacting to light. Look over here, Monty, now over here." I moved the light in each direction and he followed it with his eyes.

"Good. Now his heart and lungs." I prodded on really just to fill the frightened silence and to take charge of the situation. Monty was quiet now but looking sadly from mom to dad and to me, and back again. "Heart and lungs clear, nothing in his tummy or down below. Arms move in all directions, no fractures or dislocations, and the other leg is fine. That's why I X-rayed both. Check the pelvis and hip joint, good. We will have to check his urine for blood when he deigns to pass some. No rush, and if those are normal, we'll be all set, won't we, Monty?"

I had followed the mother through her pregnancy and delivered this, her fourth child, without any difficulty. We were comfortable with each other. Nevertheless, they both looked at me askance as I painted their little lad's legs liberally with brown balsam.

"I love that smell," I said as I finished. "Now let that dry for a few minutes, it won't take long."

"What's it for?" the mother asked.

"To protect the legs from the adhesive on the Elastoplast. You'll see." I started to hum contentedly. So far, so good, and they were interested.

"Both legs, Doctor?"

"Yes." I was enjoying this. I felt like a conjurer leading his audience up the garden path.

"At last it's dry enough now. Give me the Elastoplast please."

I took it off the nurse and applied it to the outside of his good leg length-wise down past the knee and ankle, leaving a fifteen-centimetre loop free below the sole of his foot before running it up the inside of his leg. Not so close to his bottom that he would soil it and make it dirty. Now the tensor bandage, starting at the side and wrapped firmly but not too tightly around his leg down to his ankle, cutting off the excess.

I then treated the other leg similarly, although handling the broken leg much more gently.

This is beginning to sound like a recipe, and like a recipe, it takes longer to tell than to do.

"And now the wooden blocks, if you have them."

"Will this do? I found the block of wood the cooks used to prop the kitchen window open and I broke it in two."

"Perfect." I stuck one each inside the loops of Elastoplast that I had left under each foot and covered the rough ends so they wouldn't scratch the little fellow. I could see that they were still puzzled, but I left them in the dark, still playing the conjurer, delaying the denouement.

"If Daddy will pick the little chap up and bring him to his bed, and if you bring the drip stand, Louise, I'll bring the rest of the paraphernalia."

We all walked in procession down the length of the hall until we reached the children's ward at the far end. All of the other patients were peering at us from their rooms, whispering to each other as we went past.

"Right, Daddy, put him down and let's have the drip stand at the bottom of the bed. This is going to be the tricky bit."

With a bit of difficulty, we maneuvered the stand so that the crossbar hung over the cot. Then taking two links of Elastoplast, and with the nurse holding the child's ankles up in the air, I threaded some wrapping around the wood blocks and wound the tape several turns around the old iron drip stand. Then I carefully slid the crossbar up the shaft of the stand until Monty's hips were off the bed and the length of his legs and pelvis was suspended in mid-air while his back, chest, arms, and head were resting on the mattress.

"There you are," I said with a flourish of my arms.

Dead silence.

"Now what, Doctor?" the mother said, aghast.

"A cup of coffee and a cigarette all around, I think."

My audience was not impressed.

"Well, that's it," I added lamely. Now that it was up, it did not look as impressive as it had at the Sick Kids Hospital. I looked around.

"Look, you saw how the bone ends overlapped on the X-ray? No? Well, we will go and have another look at it and I'll show you. His feet are hanging from the stand, and with his bottom off the bed, gravity will slowly and inexorably pull him down. His muscles are in spasm now, but as the pain lessens, the muscles will relax and his bottom will come down to the bed. As it does, we'll raise the bar and inch his feet further up till his bottom is off the bed again, and his thigh muscles will relax some more until the bone ends are in proper alignment."

I demonstrated weakly with my fingers. "Ends will no longer overlap and natural forces will bring them together, where a bony callous will form and they will knit back together."

"Won't he have a limp, then, Doctor?"

"No, remember he isn't a year old yet, and he won't stop growing until he is eighteen or so, by which time nature will have adjusted for everything. You'll see."

"But how will we change his diapers with that contraption?"

"You simply put one flat under his bum and the second one over the top of him. Just tuck the top one down between his legs so he doesn't pee all over the strapping."

"How will we feed him?"

"Same as always. I bet you give him a bottle in his pram when he's lying down, don't you?"

"But what about his Pablum and mashed potatoes and such? He'll choke!"

"No, he won't. There are lots of crippled people who have to be spoon-fed all their lives, aren't there, nurse?"

"Yes, I suppose so. In Valley View, the home for the disabled in Moose Jaw," the nurse replied.

Perhaps the response with a reference to the permanently disabled was not the way to go. Never mind, we'll see, I thought silently.

"And how will he sleep swinging in the breeze like that?"

"We are all adaptable. You'll be surprised. Just put a blanket over him to keep him warm and we will leave you with him for as long as you like, just call if you need anything."

I could see that Louise was not very happy with the situation, so I took her back to the X-ray room to explain in greater detail.

She still looked skeptical. "But if the Elastoplast stretches…"

"It will, but then you simply slide the crossbar up until he is suspended again. Easy. Trust me." Now I sounded like a conman.

"And what about pain relief?" she asked, still doubtful.

"Give him a teaspoonful of Tylenol and a teaspoonful of Benadryl. That's all he will need. He will relax and go to sleep with a beatific smile on his face. Just get his mom to give him a bottle of warm milk now and let her come in all day and all night if necessary. It will please the family and take a lot of work off your hands."

I crossed the yard to the suite, leaving instructions to call me if there were any problems.

The next morning after an unbroken night's sleep, I found my young patient smiling and contented—having slept intermittently but uncomplainingly, much to everybody's surprise. His mother had spent the night in there, giving him his 6 a.m.

bottle, and then had been relieved by her husband. The drip stand had to be adjusted and tied securely to the bedrail, but it was working satisfactorily, so we left it alone. His bowels had moved satisfactorily and his bladder was working well. No blood in either, much to my satisfaction. So far, so good.

Days became weeks. Not only did everyone in the hospital want to know about Monty but so did his older brothers, his cousins, and their schoolmates, and, thereafter, there was a constant traffic of people coming to see the upside-down baby, which I didn't discourage. It was good to have people seeing what we did with their money in their hospital, and it helped to give us some good publicity. Monty soon got used to his unusual view of the world, and as his family saw that he was thriving, they became less nervous and entered into the spirit of things. The general feeling was that we were doing things in our hospital and not just referring things out to the city, and that gave them confidence in all of us.

Time passed and Monty was obviously not in any pain. He allowed us to feel his legs, even squeeze them, without wincing or crying, but I was still anxious for the three weeks to pass. If we took his legs down to X-ray him and the fracture had not yet started to knit, the ends might slip into the overlap position again and we would be back to square one.

When the day arrived when I had promised to repeat the X-ray of his leg, the family was out in force all with their fingers crossed. "The films are great. Very clear." The bone ends were in alignment, as I had promised, and there was a great ball of callous around the fractured ends. I felt that we could let him out of his contraption but that we should keep the Elastoplast in place in case of any problems arising.

After another week, I allowed him to go home. As he had not really started to walk at the time he took his tumble, he wasn't going to try and walk just yet, so we let him take his time and he made steady progress. He was soon toddling around under his own steam, and further X-rays showed no evidence of kinking under the strain of his body weight. He passed his normal milestones with no real problems arising.

Years later, after I left LaFleche, I received a large, flat, stiffened envelope in the mail. It contained a photograph of Monty in his crib with his legs up in the air and a thank-you letter from the now eighteen-year-old, Grade 12 student, telling me he had won top prizes in the school sports day. Very satisfying—the photo stands on my bookcase still.

People are apt to say, "You can't win them all," to which I always reply, "By the same token, you can't lose them all either."

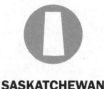

**SASKATCHEWAN**

# Dr. Paul Dhillon

*Paul Dhillon is an avid traveller with wide interests within medicine. Shortly after completing his Diploma in Tropical Medicine in London, he worked as a physician in an Ebola treatment centre in Sierra Leone. He completed his medical degree at the Royal College of Surgeons in Ireland and then completed a master's degree in disaster medicine in Italy. He was active in representing resident physicians during his family medicine residency in Saskatchewan, and in 2013 he was awarded the Canadian Medical Association Resident Leadership Award and the Murray Stalker award from the College of Family Physicians of Canada. A long-time Rotarian, he is a multiple Paul Harris Fellow. He currently practises rural and remote medicine in Canada and is a Captain with the Canadian Armed Forces 16 Field Ambulance in Regina. He currently calls Saskatchewan home with his Irish wife, Sarah.*

## Death Is Closer Here

Dying here, far from any building over two storeys, is very different than dying in the city.

Death is closer here, more intimate. The drive to work along a lonely grey road is not only marked by a yellow meridian but also by the red of roadkill. I don't remember seeing any roadkill in Regina's city centre when I was training.

In Regina, we had an incredible palliative care team to refer to, people to call when we knew that any medicine we had was not going to heal anymore. Out here, they were going to have to call me.

My first real job. Thirteen years since high school—in training, in hospitals, in books. All of a sudden at 8 a.m. tomorrow morning I would suddenly become Dr. Dhillon. Time to heal and fix. I began my first real posting as a rural physician in a small town in rural Saskatchewan. A beautiful little hospital, staff happy to see a young doctor in town, and the welcoming red and green of the local Co-op sign.

The day began innocuously enough: morning rounds at the hospital, learning about all the patients who had been handed over to my care for the next two weeks; trying to decipher other physicians' illegible writing and promising to never let mine get that bad, and failing quickly at that.

"Hello, good morning. My name is Dr. Dhillon and I'll be keeping an eye on you for the next little while until your doctor is back."

With a vague idea of what was actually happening inside each patient's body, and not a clue what was happening in their minds, I popped in from room to room as cheerful as I could be while making a list of things to check and recheck after the morning ward round was done. Thankfully, the nurses were there to handle any miscues and give me a vital, two-to-three-sentence summary of the patient and any concerns before entering into their realm with a quick knock on a half-opened door.

When I got to the last patient I was to see that morning, I found his door was closed. It was at the back corner of the hospital. It was darker.

"This is Gary, he's dying."

The nurse's tone of voice lowered, naturally, to the level we use when discussing death, just in case death was nearby and would hear and come hither to hasten the process.

"Metastatic, it was too late when he came in. Really sad story. He's still so young." She continued.

*Fuck*, I thought silently.

"Where is the primary?" I asked out loud.

"His liver, you'll see, he's completely yellow," she continued.

Thinking back, I don't know exactly how I felt when I reached for the institutionally grey doorknob. I probably felt pretty grey. They don't really tell you how you're supposed to talk to someone for the first time when all you know about them is their first name and roughly where the first cell went berserk and started its new life as a cancer that would take their life away.

I gently knocked, lighter, more gently compared to the knock for the patient who was recovering from a gall-bladder attack whom I had just chatted to.

"Hello Gary, how are you this morning?" is what I said.

"Hello, who are you?" he asked.

Within that three seconds, I had seen his distended abdomen (*ascities—check*), nasal cannula (*difficulty breathing, pressure from the abdominal fluid?*), yellow skin (*bilirubin overload*), yellow sclera (*shit… it's bad*), and dark, dark, almost-orange urine (*this is really bad, he's a great case for a medical student to see*).

All that I had been trained to think and see, diagnose, and *cure* wasn't going to help me now.

"My name is Paul and I'll be your doctor until your normal doctor comes back." I couldn't bear to say I was Dr. Dhillon. What was I going to doctor in his case?

"I'm leaving on Tuesday. Next week. To be closer to home," he said through halting inspirations.

"That's great, so that's something to look forward to then." Inside, I wondered, *Was that even appropriate to say?*

The nursing staff didn't have any new concerns, and he was eating and pain-free on his current medications, so we ended our morning chat and I went off to the clinic to finish off the rest of the day.

I couldn't stop thinking about him, though. Was there anything I could do to make him better? More comfortable? Was there anything I was missing?

As a new doctor, and still scared of missing something or making some mistake, I would do rounds twice a day. The nurses and staff probably thought it was very conscientious of me, but it was more out of fear of missing something that I shouldn't have.

Over the next week, our talks extended.

I was able to meet his family, his children. From conversations overheard while walking in the hallways, from nursing staff handovers, a picture of a life emerged. Not just a yellowed man dying in a wheelchair who couldn't breathe; a picture of a man who was battling against something completely foreign to him. A man that had his life enter the twists and turns that occur in all our lives, but in his case, the road stopped much too early.

It was a week later, on a quiet Monday morning, that I noted his birthday was the following day.

His last birthday ever.

We physicians are notoriously bad at predicting death. But I knew in this case.

Through our conversations, I had the sense that he would appreciate a birthday cake. He was a farmer before fighting the unseen cancer cells had become his full-time occupation. It could be that he had not had a proper birthday cake in years. He would have been too busy harvesting to take time for something like that.

He had time now. But not that much time.

I went quickly to the local Co-op after work. I needed a birthday cake, stat. The only cakes available were predecorated with icing designs appropriate only for an eight-year-old girl's birthday, a girl who was really, really into pink and sparkles.

How do you explain that you need a cake redecorated tonight, in the last hours the store is open, for someone who is going to die but has a birthday tomorrow, without sounding like a complete weirdo? Also, don't forget that you want to decorate the cake with small plastic farm animals to remind him of home and work and the happy times in his life.

It can't be that hard to find that sort of thing in small-town Saskatchewan at 6 p.m. on a Monday evening? Right?

Somehow, it all worked out. There remains, however, a very confused sales-counter checkout girl in a Home Hardware somewhere in Saskatchewan who is still wondering how finding small, plastic farm animals in the basement of a shop could be so exciting to the new physician in town.

On the rainy morning of his birthday, I was able to collect a number of the nurses, light some candles, and walk into his room to see a look first of confusion then surprise on his face, and then a smile that for a moment wiped the disease from the room and replaced it with pure happiness.

One of the nurses reminded him to first take off his nasal cannula blowing oxygen through to his lungs before bringing the flames close to him. *Phew.*

I left before having a chance to try the cake with him and his family, but I stuck my head in the door that afternoon. I knew, he knew, that he was leaving.

"Thanks, Doc, that was the best cake I have ever had. It was amazing."

He'll never know how those words made me feel. There was nothing years of training could have taught me to have made that situation any better for him medically. But I would like to think I made him a little happier.

His friend told me afterwards in the hallway that he was happy all day.

Then he was gone.

# Dr. Ryan Meili

*Ryan Meili splits his time between family medicine, family life, research, teaching, writing, and advocacy. He has practised in Mozambique, rural Saskatchewan, and inner-city Saskatoon. Currently, he is a family doctor at the Westside Community Clinic in Saskatoon and an assistant professor at the College of Medicine, University of Saskatchewan, where he serves as head of the Division of Social Accountability, director of the Making the Links Certificate in Global Health, and co-lead of SHARE: the Saskatchewan HIV/ AIDS Research Endeavour. He narrowly escaped leading the New Democratic Party of Saskatchewan on two occasions. His 2012 book,* A Healthy Society: How a Focus on Health Can Revive Canadian Democracy, *blends scholarship and story to point the way towards a more meaningful public discourse and has sold thousands of copies across Canada. Ryan also serves as vice-chair of the national advocacy organization, Canadian Doctors for Medicare, and is the founding director of Upstream: Institute for a Healthy Society.*

## Catch and Release

Doctors tend to remember their "saves," brushes with death or dismemberment averted—at times because of their intervention, often enough despite it—in technicolour detail. In some ways, rural physicians are the manifestation of Holden Caulfield's naive dream, the bodies catching bodies coming through the rye. It is this gatekeeper role between worlds that defines our self-image. Sure, most of our days are spent in the other gate-keeper role, determining who needs a referral to a specialist or other intervention beyond primary care, or, to paraphrase Voltaire, entertaining the patient while nature heals them.

I spent the first two or three years of my medical career as a travelling entertainer, working as a locum in rural Saskatchewan with gigs in all four corners of a province as geographically diverse as it is geometrically straightforward.

For me, it's the most dramatic cases that first spring to mind. Transporting patients with massive myocardial infarctions or flash pulmonary edema down bad roads in deep, dark winter, feeling like Santa Claus "bagging all the way." Delivering a thirty-two-weeker in a nursing station on a reserve while my colleague stabilizes a seizing two-year-old in the next room. The surprise of discovering that a woman didn't lose the fractured and purple foot we'd wrapped up after she was found struck by a vehicle and left in the ditch at thirty below on New Year's Eve. Packaging a young man with two fractured femurs and a head injury for transport to the city after he was run over by an RCMP truck on a reserve. Little miracles of a bit of good medicine and a lot of luck.

Perhaps the most memorable of all was the sweet miracle of Entwhistle, the closest thing I've seen to a resurrection. A man in his mid-forties was carried into the emergency room in this small, eastern Saskatchewan, potash-mining town. He'd been found unconscious in his garage, and on the Glasgow Coma Scale—the measurement we use to tell how conscious or unconscious a patient is—he scored a three, the lowest score out of a possible fifteen. Even with a painful sternal rub (knuckles pressed hard against the breastbone), he didn't move a muscle, twitch an eye, or make a sound. There was no history of trauma, nothing unusual about the past twenty-four hours, except that he'd had a few drinks with his buddies over cards. His family reported that he had diabetes that was well controlled with oral medications and was otherwise healthy as far as they knew. On examination, aside from being completely comatose, he was well. He was hemodynamically stable, meaning his blood pressure and heart rate were normal, as was his breathing. Despite this, he was completely out of reach.

I was more than a bit baffled by this presentation, and my mind went back to an experience in medical school when on an elective in rural Zambia. A skinny old man with long dreadlocks was laid out on the little grey cot that served as the emergency room. He, too, was dead to the world, completely unresponsive to voice or pain. My preceptor, an experienced internist who'd been visiting the region for many years, had seen this before. "I have no idea what's in the homebrew, but we see someone like this every once in a while. Sugar seems to work." And did it ever! She gave him an injection of IV dextrose, a high-concentration sugar solution. He sat up like a bolt, said he had to pee, and ran out of the hospital. We never saw him again.

With that story in mind, I checked the glucose of the patient in Entwhistle. It was perfectly normal, even a touch on the high side. Still, I thought it couldn't hurt and tried the same trick with an injection of dextrose. Just like his Zambian counterpart, to the amazement of his family, the skeptical nurses, and me, too, he sat up straight and started talking as though nothing was out of the ordinary. After a few minutes of pure lucidity, alert and oriented, explaining in detail the events of the night before, he started to drift off again. Within moments, he was as unreachable as before. We repeated the dextrose, which woke him again and, despite his diabetes, started him on a regular drip of the same and made arrangements to ship him to Regina for further investigations.

I've asked a few fellow doctors since and have even done some research to try to find out why that worked. I've yet to find anyone who could give me a clear explanation, though it may be explained by neuroglycopenia, meaning different levels of glucose in the brain and the rest of the body under certain circumstances.

The only cases we remember more clearly than those we catch are those we don't. On my office wall I don't have my MD hanging. I have a framed transfer note that was never sent, a note about the first patient who died under my care. I was a medical student working in a rural hospital in Mozambique. At around 7 p.m., on July 8, 2002, a man in his mid-forties was brought into the emergency room by his family members. They reported that he'd been complaining of headache and had been vomiting since the night before. At nine that morning, he tried to get out of bed and fell to the ground; he'd been unconscious and unable to move one side of his body since. His blood pressure was through the roof, he was paralyzed on one side, and he had a fever. Not understanding at that point in my training that malaria could cause a stroke, I didn't start quinine immediately the way we did with most patients with a high fever. This meant it wasn't started until a couple of hours later when we were able to track down the doctor on call. God only knows if it would have made any difference in such a severe case, but it should have been started right away. The patient never recovered consciousness and was dead by morning.

I've thought through that case a hundred times since. Thought about Berto, the often-drunk-at-work health agent who sanguinely told me not to bother with the transfer note. "You can't save everyone." Thought about how I shouldn't have been in that emergency room in the first place. Thought about the fact that if I wasn't there, no one else was. Thought about how even if doing things differently wouldn't change the outcome, I still wish I'd done things differently.

In the winter of 2009, I spent a week in Spirit River, a mill town on the forest fringe of northeast Saskatchewan. I was working again as a rural locum, this time in a stable practice with a group of really good physicians. I worked days in the clinic and during the evenings I went exploring around town and watched bad movies I'd rented at the convenience store.

On Friday afternoon, just before my weekend of call, Betty Trotchie came in with her husband. They lived a half-hour out of town on the farm where they'd raised their kids, now grown up and spread out around the country with kids of their own. They'd both quit smoking a few years earlier, but decades of tobacco use had left their mark. Betty had a long history of chronic obstructive pulmonary disease, often referred to as emphysema, which occasionally got bad enough to require antibiotics, and once before she'd needed to come into the hospital.

She always had a cough, but that Friday it was a little heavier than usual, and she said she was "coughing up more junk." When I listened to her lungs, there were crackling sounds at the bottom, just like you'd expect in someone with COPD. I decided to check her oxygen saturation, which turned out to be around 85 per cent. Had it been above 90 per cent, I might have just sent her home with antibiotics, but I thought it best to admit her instead. We discussed the possibility of her going to Saskatoon—the nearest tertiary care centre—for more intensive management. They didn't want to do this, and in the same conversation we discussed end-of-life care. She and her husband were quite clear about their wishes for her treatment, and that included not wanting to have a tube to assist with her breathing.

So we kept her there at the rural hospital, starting oxygen, IV antibiotics, and other medications to help with her breathing. She settled into her room, the one in-patient bed in the whole hospital, and her husband went to the farm to get her a few things for her stay.

One of the local physicians, Dr. Weldon, had invited me over for supper that evening. Once I'd written up all the admission orders and Betty was settled in, I went over to his house. It was on the opposite end of town from the hospital, which in a town that size was less than a ten-minute walk away. Dr. Weldon had come to Spirit River thirty years previous with three colleagues from med school. He was the last one from the original group, and had stuck it out through good times with stable colleagues and through the rough times, too, when they were down to two docs and being on call was essentially always. He'd lived through the ups and downs of a single-industry town, living and dying the trials and travails of his patients and neighbours as one of them, not just a visiting hired hand. For his kids, this wasn't a town their dad had decided to come and serve, it was the only home they'd known. His patients were their hockey teammates and elementary school teachers, their friends' grandmothers. We talked Saskatchewan politics, medical education, changing small-town life, and the somewhat bleak and open-ended question of the future of medicine in towns like Spirit River. We chatted a bit about Betty as well; she was his colleague's patient, but he knew the family well.

I checked in on Betty again that evening. Her breathing had become more difficult, and despite medications and an even higher oxygen concentration, her oxygen saturation was falling into the low eighties. I saw her again first thing Saturday morning and a few more times throughout the day, and left instructions to be called in with any changes to her condition.

At noon on Saturday, her husband asked if he should call in the family, including a daughter in Calgary, a good ten hours away. I told him I couldn't be sure, but it might be a good idea. It was a good thing she came, as her mother's condition only continued to deteriorate. By Saturday night, she was asleep and barely responsive. At 6 a.m. on Sunday morning the nurse on duty called me in to tell me Betty had died. I went in to see her and sat with the family awhile. They were extremely kind to me, a stranger, and thankful for the care their mother had received. They seemed to think it was a good death, the kind of passing she would have wanted.

Patients die. They're supposed to. Doctors hang around sick people. If the doctor's any good, the sicker they are, the more the doctor hangs around, and, ultimately, the more patients they lose. Me, I look forward to someday being a patient well lost.

And for the most part, Betty's passing *was* exactly what most of us would want. She was joking and laughing one day, and had her family gathered around to see her off the next. She made up her own mind about what needed to be done, died close to home, and avoided a potentially prolonged and invasive hospitalization.

But let's face it, it's not that clear-cut. Her last hours were peaceful, but were they premature? There's a pretty good chance that if she'd gone to town, she'd still be alive today. And there's a pretty good chance that if I'd thought she was going to die that weekend, I could have convinced her to take that trip. We talk of, and strive for, informed consent, but so much is dependent on what the attending physician thinks is likely or preferable. The consent of the patient is only as informed as the physician who seeks it. Try as I might, and I've wracked my brains over Betty's case, there's nothing about her presentation that made her stand out from dozens of other people I'd hospitalized with exacerbations of COPD.

Yet, on some level, it feels like rather than trying desperately to catch her, we stepped aside a little too easily, let her go too quietly into that good night. I'm not sure the family, or even Betty, would agree. Not all the bodies want to be caught.

Still, it nags at me.

Of course, everyone goes over the edge eventually, but that's little solace when your job is to delay the drop. This, to me, is the wonder and the horror of rural medicine. There are EMTs and nursing staff, UpToDate (an online resource for physicians), and the on-call service in the nearest big centre, but despite all of this the decisions land on a lone doc over and over again. What to keep, what to send? Today, it's a pneumothorax and you've only practised chest tubes on pigs, tomorrow a dislocated shoulder that just won't reduce. Every day, you're making it up as you go along, hoping you know how to catch those you can, and even harder, hoping you know which ones to let fall.

On Monday morning, bags already packed and the key to the locum apartment left with the charge nurse, I came in to finish up some charting and hand things over to Dr. Weldon. I told him about the other in-patient admitted the day before, and matter-of-factly about Betty's passing, a physician-to-physician transaction of information. "Mrs. Trotchie died Sunday morning."

"Really? Oh my God!" he replied, with a look of real surprise that caught me off guard. It was not the detached, professional response I'm used to. He looked shocked and disappointed, as though I was talking about a member of his own family. He may very well have been asking himself, "What if I'd been on call instead?" I was left wondering the same thing.

I'm not a rural physician anymore. I work in the inner city, a place I often describe as "so urban it's rural," and while the day-to-day practice reflects that, the tertiary backup around the corner changes everything. I've been in my neighbourhood long enough to feel some of what Dr. Weldon felt when one of my patients dies. Still, there's something about the anonymity of the city, and the sharing of practice with so many others, that dilutes that spooky, exhilarating feeling of waiting alone in a wheat field.

**SASKATCHEWAN**

# Dr. Kevin Wasko

*Kevin Wasko grew up in Eastend, Saskatchewan. After graduating from high school in Eastend, he attended Dalhousie University in Halifax, Nova Scotia, earning a bachelor of arts in political science. He then obtained a master of arts in political science from the University of Calgary. Kevin spent time in medical administration with the Cypress Health Region in Swift Current, Saskatchewan, and then worked in the office of the Minister of Health of Saskatchewan prior to attending medical school at the University of Calgary, where he received his MD in 2011. He completed his residency in family medicine through the University of Saskatchewan's rural training site in Swift Current, where he now practises full-scope family medicine, works emergency shifts, practises low-risk maternity care, and lives with his wife Kylie and children Jade and Henry. A self-professed news junkie, he also enjoys running, skiing, and curling in his spare time.*

## A Rural Return

Eastend, Saskatchewan, a quaint and idyllic community nestled in a valley of rolling hills at the east end of the Cypress Hills of southwest Saskatchewan, is my hometown. A community of less than five hundred people, it has attracted a diverse population of cattle ranchers, grain farmers, artists, writers, and paleontology enthusiasts. My roots in that community extend back for generations. In fact, all four of my grandparents have spent their entire lives in that community, and it is home to my parents as well.

It was in the sixth grade that I decided unwaveringly that I was going to become a doctor one day and treat the people of Eastend. I remember being congratulated on my goal in a placating sort of way. Rarely did someone in rural Saskatchewan grow up to actually become a physician. Even if I was not fully aware of that fact at the time, I certainly am now. I do not have the hard numbers and statistics, but the percentage of rural kids who grow up to become doctors is less than kids from the city. There are multiple reasons for this, ranging from a lack of mentorship to parental education levels to financial resources and more.

While my initial goal of treating and caring for the people of Eastend was steadfastly absolute in the sixth grade, my resolution seemed to wane with the more education I accumulated. There were certainly times when I was convinced I would never become a physician at all. Once that goal was all but assured upon admission to medical school, the thought of returning to Eastend to work was not even on my radar. It wasn't until I neared completion of my family medicine residency that I pondered providing an itinerant clinic in Eastend.

The medical services in Eastend have certainly changed. When I was growing up, there was a sole general practitioner who worked in Eastend. He was a loud and, at times, brash South African doctor who was larger than life but cared for that community wholeheartedly. He was one of the last holdouts of the era when solo country doctors cared for their communities, on a 24/7 basis, and practised full-scope family medicine and then some. Indeed, he was what I grew up thinking a doctor was and should be. Undoubtedly, he shaped my approach towards my own practice and work ethic as a physician. When he passed away after twenty-two years in the community, the people of Eastend found themselves without a primary care provider.

A solo GP from South Africa was recruited and left within a year of coming. Eventually, a primary health care model was introduced at the health centre in town, a facility that includes long-term care patients, a small outpatient department, respite beds, and lab and X-ray services. Clinics were set up with nurse practitioners and visiting family physicians based out of Maple Creek, located one hour northwest of Eastend.

Because I still have strong links to the community, I knew there was dissatisfaction with the care people were receiving. There were often inconsistencies with care providers and ultimately care plans. This was not the fault of the providers but inevitable given the set-up. The larger issue seemed to be a mistrust of the system, and I could see that people longed to trust a care provider like they had once trusted that venerable physician who cared for them for over two decades. I was not convinced that could ever really be achieved, but the challenge appealed to me, as did the desire to care for my fellow compatriots.

In August of this past year, I found myself realizing my sixth-grade ambition. One month out of residency, I held my first clinic in Eastend. I joined the primary health care team there and committed to commute one and a half hours each way to provide clinical services every Wednesday.

The first day at the clinic in Eastend seemed somewhat surreal. It was hard to believe that my long and arduous road to becoming a physician had brought me right back to where I had started. I knew all the staff and although there was comfort in familiarity, it also evoked nervousness about how they would approach my role as a leader of the health care team.

I entered the facility thinking it was one I knew well and indeed I did. However, with the lens I now looked through, things appeared different. As I walked into the small outpatient treatment room, I had a flashback to passing out while having a skin biopsy performed on me as a teenager. It was a story I later related to a young patient while removing a skin lesion. I told it with the intention of putting her at ease but quickly realized it may have done the opposite.

As I looked over my patient list for the day, I was reassured that all of the slots had been completely filled. Although I thought most people would likely be fine with seeing me as a physician, there had been a nagging in the back of my mind that people might rather see someone with whom they were less personally familiar. I worried that they might not take me seriously as a new physician. It also made me nervous to see certain names. While I worried about people not wanting to see me, I never contemplated not wanting to see friends and distant relatives for certain medical ailments.

As time has passed, I have quickly become accustomed to providing medical care to people I have known my entire life. This is something that most physicians don't experience. I appreciate that I know the patient's context without having to ask. I know their marital situation, if they have just recently lost a spouse or parent, where they work, their children, and their financial means. I care for multiple generations of patients within the same families. Being from the community, I also know the familial connections. As a result, I sometimes have greater insight into their family history than they do themselves. Every face is familiar and for the most part that puts us both at ease.

In my short time in practice, I have come to realize the major impact that my new role holds in the lives of these people. I picked up a new onset of unstable angina and my prompt referral resulted in an urgent coronary bypass surgery. By picking up a colon cancer in its early stages, another patient underwent bowel resection surgery before it became metastatic. These catches were gratifying and perhaps more so because of the preceding personal connection with the patients. At the same time, the realization that I could very well be missing major diagnoses in these people was equally impactful. It has perhaps made me a more prudent physician.

All the while, I have also had to become accustomed to practicing in such a rural and remote part of the country. As a physician practicing hours away from the tertiary centres, one is faced with different challenges and obstacles. Geography, the finances of the patient, and ease of travel factor into decision-making processes. Tertiary care is nearly four hours away, in Regina, and it is nearly five hours to Saskatoon. I am the only physician working in the clinic at any time and acute care services are twenty minutes down the road in Shaunavon. This contrasts with my experience in Swift Current, where I practise in a clinic with eight other physicians in a community with a regional hospital staffed by core specialists. From there, tertiary care in Regina is two hours away on a divided highway.

Rural physicians must comfortably practise to their full range of ability so that patients can, where possible, receive care in their home communities. I find that during my days in Eastend I am more likely to solve the problem myself and prescribe medications that I am fairly confident my specialist colleagues would prescribe if I referred them on. For instance, while I might seek a dermatologist's input for a case of severe psoriasis for my patient in Swift Current, I am more likely to initiate methotrexate myself for the Eastend patient. Indeed, for the patient from Eastend, a four-hour drive to Regina for a ten-minute consult is a greater ordeal, especially during winter in Saskatchewan. I don't think this means I am providing a differential in care but that I am taking the patient's context into account.

It is for the reason of understanding the rural context that I have incorporated learners into my clinic in Eastend. I now have either a family medicine resident or a medical student from the University of Saskatchewan with me every time I work there. The time that medical learners spend in Eastend will expose them to what rural medicine really looks like. It is the hope that this exposure might inspire them to serve rural communities in the future. Even if they ultimately end up practicing as a specialist in an urban centre, they will have a better understanding of where these patients come from and the burden they have assumed to travel vast distances to access medical care.

Few people can truly say they grew up to fulfill their sixth-grade aspiration. Not only have I done that but I also couldn't be happier about the choices that have led me back to where I started.

Robert C. Bowman said, "Physicians who are drawn to rural practice want to make a difference in peoples' lives and want to have a respected position where you care for a town and the town cares for you." This statement summarizes the major reasons why I chose to become a physician in the first place, and I feel humbled that I am able to live out that goal now.

**SASKATCHEWAN**

# Dr. Ankit Kapur with Dr. Puneet Kapur

*Originally from Milton, Ontario, the Kapur brothers have made their homes in Saskatchewan. Ankit is living the rural life in the North with his two dogs and his partner Julia, a fellow family resident. Meanwhile, Puneet enjoys the challenges of his five-year emergency medicine training in Saskatoon. With Puneet's prior life as a computer scientist and Ankit's background in international humanitarian relief, the brothers have combined their skills to focus on using technology to improve health care in remote communities.*

## Making Mistakes

Joy was the feeling with which I started my family medicine residency on July 1, 2014, in La Ronge, Saskatchewan. It was a dream come true—almost a decade of my life had been spent training to one day be able to work as a rural physician and now I finally had that chance.

Fear, however, was the emotion that dominated my first few weeks, if not months, of work. All those years of training supposedly prepared me to care for people, to preserve life and defend against illness. But I was terrified of making errors, of hurting someone with my ignorance or arrogance, of not knowing enough to catch a problem early. I tried to read up on everything I encountered; I snuck to the back room during patient appointments to look up information; I reviewed matters with my supervising physician often and in detail. But I knew it with statistical certainty that I would eventually make a significant mistake—it was only a matter of time.

Time, of course, is the constant enemy of medicine. We often have too little, or things are taking too long. Such is the case with medical training as well. It takes a great deal of time to become an experienced clinician, and we often have too little time to get all our work done. This leads to an almost cliché situation of a junior trainee, overworked and underexperienced. And so I found myself, green and tired, on my second on-call shift of residency.

Our emergency department had nine beds and was staffed with a nurse and a physician, and the day I joined them as a resident doctor, the title still felt awkward and heavy. Being July in the north of Canada, the sun stayed up late, happily warming the lakes and forests until almost 11 p.m. The people stayed out late as well—walking, fishing, and generally enjoying the weather—and as you would imagine, with all that activity, some of these denizens found their way into our little emergency department.

It was a busy night and I could see the attending physician was happy to have me around to help. I was eager to please and keen to get as much experience as quickly as possible, so I welcomed every additional consult, task, and call. By 10 p.m., fourteen hours into my shift, I finally started feeling the toll of nonstop activity. I started to want the pace to slow, to be able to clear off my to-do list a little, and to maybe even take a little break.

It was then that I got a call from one of the nurses at a remote northern outpost. She was concerned about a young woman who came in with a friend. Both were previously well, they both had a few days' history of vomiting and diarrhea, both had fevers in the 38–39°C range, and both had reported eating out the day the symptoms started. I listened to this presentation for a few minutes while the nurse continued to describe system by system every finding—unable to parse the relevant from the benign. I listened with decreasing interest as my mind had already selected acute gastroenteritis as the most likely diagnosis for both. As the presentation went on, I could see my emergency department filling up, and the list of tasks in front of me seemed to be growing on its own, so finally I interrupted, as I had seen so many physicians do before, and I asked a few questions, in an almost perfunctory way, regarding neck stiffness and chemical exposure to ensure I had not missed an important diagnosis. I felt good having thought broadly about the diagnosis, I was proud to have considered other causes when I was sure others might not have, and I confidently told the nurse on the phone to let them go home with Tylenol and instructions regarding the management of gastroenteritis--and that if things got worse, they should come back.

After reviewing with my attending physician, my surety was solidified; this was definitely gastroenteritis and I almost regretted even having wasted so much time listening to a long, drawn-out story. In my inexperience, what I had missed was not anything clinical; rather, I lacked the subtle art of listening to tone and feeling that comes with experience and not textbooks.

I missed the nurse's apprehensions and worry regarding these patients—the one in particular. I mistook her painstaking case report as poor clinical communication, but I missed that this was an attempt to communicate her concern. I missed her fear that this case was so similar to that of other people from the community who had recently become very sick and passed away. What I missed was pretty much the most important stuff.

Looking back, these errors should have been expected. While I took tremendous effort to guard against diagnostic and therapeutic errors, the reality is most medical errors happen because of poor communication. Whether it is at hand-over between shifts, during the transfer of patient care, or during a simple phone call, the data shows consistently how we communicate is the largest source of medical mistakes.

The next time I heard about these patients, one had gotten better, but the one who the nurse had been concerned about had gotten much worse. The day following my phone call, the patient had come back to the nursing station extremely short of breath and a Shock Trauma Air Rescue Society (STARS) air ambulance was tasked to transport her to Saskatoon. Once on board, though, she seemed to improve drastically—the therapeutic effect of flight I guess. Markedly improved, the STARS team changed plans and instead brought her to the nearest hospital, La Ronge.

Once in La Ronge, things changed course again. The patient became more unstable and the respiratory distress (her difficulty breathing) became so pronounced she required intubation. Once she had the tube in her trachea and a ventilator attached, STARS made its way back to La Ronge to courier the patient this time all the way to Saskatoon, where she was placed in an intensive care unit and cared for by a team that consisted of my brother, Puneet, an emergency medicine resident.

In the days and weeks to follow, I would communicate with the nurse I spoke with, the attending physicians, and Puneet. I would come to find that although I did not clinically miss any relevant facts, I had alienated the nurse who felt she hadn't been heard—I didn't understand why she had called and I didn't understand her worries. I came to learn that although I could not have anticipated the diagnosis, the other more experienced physicians were aware of other similar cases in the last few months and as such had a much lower threshold before which they would evacuate the patient. From my brother I learned how medically challenging the patient had become and how much of an unknown she was, even with all the testing they had done in the big city.

Communication with all of the parties involved was also uniquely different. With the nurse, the discourse was centred on liability and identifying who had made a mistake—she was worried she would be blamed for any negative outcome. Our relationship lacked trust and familiarity right from the beginning and it negatively affected our ability to communicate. With the physician group, I was the worried party. Although I listened and incorporated their advice, the overwhelming concern I had was that I would be blamed and an error on my side would be identified as the cause of this patient's poor outcome. I was new in residency and I didn't want to be known as unskilled or incompetent. I took solace in the fact that STARS had also felt she was stable. I defended my clinical decision by referencing the friend who had gotten much better, and all in all I tried my best to justify my choices.

But with my brother there was true communication. We obviously both knew each other and trusted each other's abilities. We were both trainees, and we were both confused by the case and both clinically curious. We spent hours reviewing films, blood work, progress notes; we talked openly about diagnoses and we critically critiqued each other's management.

In the end, the patient was identified as having a rare illness carried by mouse feces containing a hantavirus. It was one of the first times this had appeared this far north in Saskatchewan and it was an atypical presentation at first. Things were stacked against even the greatest diagnostician figuring out what was wrong during that initial phone call.

It is undeniable, though, that had I been a better listener, had my communication been more open, and had there been more trust and familiarity between myself and the outpost nurse, that patient may have been receiving better care sooner. As I compared the quality of the communication between the nurse and

I to that between me and Puneet, the differences were stark. I realized that to communicate well, we must first take the time to know who we are in communication with. We must first develop trust, and then we must be prepared to listen—even to the things not said.

As I develop as a physician, I have to now try to always prioritize how I communicate and listen. And to do this, I now focus on trust; trust has become the first thing I give, and the first thing I try to earn, in all my clinical encounters—it is the very bedrock of all true communication.

Regardless of my efforts, though, error is inevitable—fear and terror will accompany each error—these are immutable truths. But I also know when these things come to pass, I can always trust my older brother for a little help.

**ALBERTA**

# Dr. Anna-Kristen Siy

*Anna-Kristen Siy is a rural family physician and family-practice anesthetist. Home is wherever her car is parked, and her trunk contains emergency airway equipment, snowshoes, and a cast-iron frying pan. She thinks too much about etymology, international development, and theology, and too little about the location of her house keys. Despite growing up a city girl, Anna's love for rural and remote medicine finds her chasing meteor showers in the dead of winter, teaching medical students in southwest Uganda or inner-city Calgary, figuring out antibiotic coverage for coyote blood exposures, and changing far too many punctured car tires between hikes. She learns the art of medicine from remarkable mentors and colleagues. She learns the art of living from her patients.*

## Darkest Day

He's dead. His daughter found him, swinging from the porch rafters.

Three days ago, she miscarried. Today, she cut him down, sawing through the rope with a cleaver, tearing at it with her hands, burying her palms in his chest until the ambulance arrived.

"Buy me some smokes," he told his wife, an hour earlier. She went. And he was alone.

The chart was hefty. Decades of hospital visits, clinic appointments, occasional admissions with blood work and drugs and attempts at trying to find whatever it was underlying his pain. Opioids, antidepressants, antiepileptics indicated for neuropathic pain, topical compounds costing $10 a gram—everything had been prescribed.

*"Patient will not take medications from Dr,"* read the home care notes. *"He will take one pill and then say that no one is helping him and throw them out."*

"Every time he comes home from the hospital, he's angry," his daughter said, sobbing, "He came home yesterday and said that the doctors were useless and he just wanted to sleep."

"Oh, it's Jonathan," said my nurse as the paramedics wheeled him in. We hooked him up to the monitors, placed pads on the hollow of his chest, my hand against his yellowing, cooling skin where his femoral pulse would have been.

Mike leaned his weight in with every compression, and the absurdity of the blood pressure readings, super-physiologically hypertensive, higher than Jonathan would have ever known in life, sent a ripple of tense laughter through us even as we pulled the curtains and shut the doors, knowing his family would soon be here.

Pulse check. No rhythm on the monitor, no life beneath my hand. It had been one hour since his daughter started CPR. It had been two hours since his wife left the house. The bruises were blossoming across his thin skin. A faint indentation still circled his throat.

I called the code. Time of death: 12:12.

"Why won't anybody help me?" he asked me yesterday, in exam room 3. "I'm tired of all of you trying to tell me nothing's wrong."

"I'm sorry," I said, "I know you're in pain. I want to help. I don't know if I can make it better today, but I want to help."

Even so, the irritation rose as I examined and listened and assessed, as he accused me of first just trying to give him pain medications and ignoring his symptoms, and later of refusing to treat his pain. I wrote him a prescription. He tore it in half and turned his back to me, hobbling on his cane out to the parking lot.

"Don't be bothered," said my nurse, "that's just his way."

## The Mermaid

0237 hours. The phone summons me from my cocoon of hospital blankets. First year of residency, first night alone in-house in this rural hospital, cortisol runs high as I flit down to emergency.

I pick up the chart and read: "10 weeks pregnant, bleeding. No fetal heartbeat on Doppler."

As I enter the room, she is poised on the examining table, all angles and edges, seemingly younger than her years. Dark eyes appraise me. Her voice is quiet and her answers are terse, though not unfriendly. I examine her. Her cervix is closed, there is no active bleeding, her vitals are reassuring, and nothing is particularly tender.

In the radiology witching hour, I have only my own hands at my disposal. With an unceremonious glob of ultrasound gel, I direct the probe through her bladder to her uterus. And there, circled in white endometrium, the fetus reposes like a mermaid in the amnion, and there, between gills—no, ribs—flutters its heart.

"She's alive. Oh thank God, she's alive."

I am so engrossed with generating a clear image that her voice startles me back into the room. Tension melts from her shoulders, tears stream from her eyes. Even as she apologizes, I reassure her, delighted to offer such deep comfort through these staid rituals of care.

I arrange formal ultrasound follow-up, give careful discharge instructions, and then bask in the reflection of her hope. After a week of disabling strokes and metastatic cancers, I am inclined to let counter-transference be damned. Her joy is my joy. I grin despite fatigue and wish her well as she calls for a ride home.

Three days later, a chart in the queue catches my eye: "10 weeks pregnant and bleeding, just had ultrasound."

I update myself. Her physical exam remains reassuring and she is afebrile and pain-free, but she continues to spot. Swabs from last visit are pending. My pager interjects. It is radiology.

I feel viscerally unwell when I return. I open my mouth and hear my own words, sharp and cruel.

"There might be something wrong with the baby's genes. Down's syndrome or maybe another type of abnormality. There are tests we can do to find out what is wrong, if something is wrong, but they have to be done in the city. I'm so sorry," I say.

"It's okay. God has a plan," she says. "There's a purpose to all of this." She is undecided about genetic testing but is confident she wants to continue the pregnancy regardless.

I am slightly envious of the comfort she clearly draws from her faith. My own beliefs are nebulous these days. I assure her she has time to make decisions and leave a note for her family doctor.

•••

My last day of the rotation involves pie and ice cream. An hour before my final parting, buoyed by goodwill and glucose, I scavenge the charts yet to be seen.

"16 weeks pregnant, leaking fluid, amniocentesis yesterday."

The ultrasound and amniocentesis report is damning. The diagnosis is pending, but the prognosis is clear: "Fetal demise expected before thirty weeks gestation."

She has had an extensive discussion with medical genetics. She understands the dismal prognosis. She knows her options. She grasps the risks of continuing the pregnancy.

"I know that I'm going to miscarry," she says, "but she's alive right now. I couldn't live with myself if I killed her. Does that make sense?"

I hesitate. "I'm not sure there's one right answer. You need to do what you believe is right."

She relaxes slightly. Her hands unclench and move to her knees.

"The nurse at the outpost couldn't find a heartbeat today, and there's been more blood. Am I miscarrying?"

The nitrazine swab is negative. Her cervix is closed.

"Do you want me to look for a heartbeat?"

I sweep the beam across her uterus. For the first time in my life, I find myself hoping for stillness. For closure.

The mermaid swims, its back to my probe, pointedly ignoring my entreaties. Four chambers dance in the field. Two fists flail out defiantly.

I shut off the screen.

Salt streams from her eyes as she lies there on the table, and all I can do is wordlessly place a hand on her shoulder.

"I don't know what to do. She's still my baby."

I pull up a chair. I hand her a towel. She wipes off the gel and pulls down her shirt but stays supine. And she talks.

She talks about what she believes and why, how she went from a string of abusive relationships and addictions to her church, a happy marriage, and two kids at home.

"And that's why I can't hurt her," she says. "I couldn't forgive myself if I took away what life she has left."

"You need to do what you feel is right," I say haltingly. "I believe some of the same things as you, and I wouldn't fault you for either decision. But I understand why you're choosing this."

She nods.

"I wish I knew why this is happening to you."

"It doesn't matter," she says. "Bad things happen. God lets them sometimes."

"Not that I can speak for God, but I think He wouldn't mind if you were angry at Him," I say. I am angry, anyhow, on her behalf.

"I couldn't be. How could I be angry at someone who's done so much for me already?"

She smiles when I tell her I admire her faith. We lapse into silence again.

The idea has occurred to me repeatedly in the last ten minutes, but it now seems opportune. "This is, well, unorthodox, but, would you want me to pray with you?"

"Please."

I come from a faith tradition of timid prayers, a Calvinistic sort of petition that is afraid to speak confidently or specifically in light of a predetermined universe. But I have parted ways with that particularly cold branch of theology, and my additional sense of injustice emboldens me. I speak for this courageous woman. I speak for the mermaid. I speak for love and hope and comfort in the face of despair.

And somehow, something shifts in the room. Somewhere in my barrage of words a levee breaks and joy floods into the tears. And with a final "Amen," we are laughing. She is speaking of the goodness of God, and I, in awe of her strength and compassion, can only agree.

She deigns to thank me on her way out. I shake my head. I am the one who should be grateful.

• • •

Today, I check the clinic notes from afar. The fetal heartbeat was absent at her last prenatal visit. Ultrasound confirmed intrauterine fetal demise.

My sorrow is only a shadow, I know. My hope and my anxiety, my joy and now my grief are anemic ghosts of my patient's experience. Yet I feel honoured to have witnessed her vulnerability and dignity, to have been humbled by her resilience, to have walked alongside her for the briefest of moments.

I struggle to speculate on the nature of souls; much less what defines life or personhood. But I know this much: the mermaid was loved as dearly as anyone has ever been loved.

I pray for her mother still.

**ALBERTA**

# Dr. Kristine Woodley

*Kristine Woodley has always been a rural doc at heart and practises the mantra of work hard, play hard. She completed her undergraduate studies at Laurentian University and received her medical degree from the Northern Ontario School of Medicine in her hometown of Sudbury in 2011. Since graduating in 2013 from the University of Calgary Rural Alberta South Family Medicine Program, she has been a locum physician in a variety of rural Alberta communities. Kristine now resides and practises in Pincher Creek with her spouse Marcus and their cat Stella Artois. She looks forward to practising in both Canada and Ireland in the future in order to spend time with her international family.*

## 100-Year Flood

The Alberta floods of 2013 caused a rise of mixed emotions in all those affected. As a second-year family medicine resident, thrilled to be saying "it's my last day of residency," I thought my little taste of a flood in High River would just be another great story to add to the many I experienced there.

But the waters kept rising.

It's still a great story, although the greatness lies in a different place than I would have expected.

June 20 was an exciting day—the completion of ten years of medical training that provided me the opportunity to meet countless interesting people, gain amazing skills, and travel across Canada. Onwards to the next adventures!

Unfortunately, June 20, 2013, also became a day of shock, change, and, at times, fear. When the water began rising in the aptly named town of High River in the early morning hours, I had no idea that my last day of residency would no longer be remembered as such but instead as the day that southern Alberta faced off with Mother Nature.

On the eve of the flood it rained, it rained a lot. Not more than I have seen in the past, but it was still a good amount. Prior to this, I had never been in or witnessed a flood before; nor had I lived in southern Alberta long enough to be wary of the month of June and the heavy downpours that could come.

I spent the early morning oblivious to the rising waters.

As the water rose around the clinic, we took pictures and I was once again told, "It isn't called High River for nothing!" When it was finally decided that it was time to shut down shop, I headed towards the hospital to work in the Low Risk Maternity Clinic. As I turned into the downtown, I drove into a wall of water. I managed to turn around and slowly began realizing this was more than we were expecting. I tried calling both the clinic and my fiancé, who was asleep in our apartment across the street from the hospital, but phones were down. I watched in naive awe as people attempted to drive out of the downtown area.

It was chaotic, to put it mildly.

Not sure that it was the right thing to do, I parked my graduation gift, a Subaru, on some dry land, assuming that the water would never get to it. I hid my iPad under the front seat, nice and dry and out of view from any potential thief. I pulled on my rubber boots, which luckily were in the back seat. As I alternatively walked, jogged, and mostly sloshed through the water towards the hospital and my apartment, I stopped a few times and just looked around, dumbfounded by what I was seeing.

I realized later that I hadn't seen anything yet.

In the next fifteen minutes, I made it home, asked my fiancé to get our belongings out of the basement, grabbed a pair of running shoes, and hitched a ride in the box of a pickup to the hospital across the river I used to call a street.

Now don't assume my fiancé was a fan of me leaving him. He was not impressed. He had as much experience as I did with floods—more specifically, none.

Unfortunately, by the time I realized how bad things were getting, there was no crossing that river to get back to him. I am eternally grateful that he is an amazing man who respects my uncontrollable urge to rush into the chaos rather than run from it. When crisis strikes, many people run towards safety, which sounds like the reasonable thing to do. As physicians and many other health care professionals, we tend to run headfirst towards it.

The next few hours were spent sand bagging and helping triage the patients that were in hospital. There were moments of frustration as we watched the waters racing past; venting that there seemed to be no help getting to us. There were helicopters flying overhead, and many of us assumed they were news stations recording the madness we were living, angering us. Then we saw a person dangling from a rope below a helicopter. That's when it really hit home…this was bad, and it wasn't just a small part of town that had become a raging river.

Throughout the day there were many moments of panic and anxiety. Communication was coming in to us that a storm surge was potentially on its way, bringing another two or more metres of water. My fiancé was across the street and I knew he didn't have two metres to stay dry. Our phones were down. I didn't know if he was still okay and my mind began playing tricks on me. I began to really worry, to the point of it affecting my focus.

I am so thankful for a nurse, a friend who helped me take a few breaths and regroup. The unknown, combined with a fierce desire to keep your loved ones safe, can have an amazing emotional impact, one I had never experienced before. Many others I spoke to afterwards experienced exactly the same feelings that day, as they couldn't find their children, spouses, and parents.

Despite all of this, there were some amazing and encouraging moments. Everyone worked together to keep the High River Hospital literally above water. Although we couldn't keep the water from entering the hospital's main level, we were able to work in teams to keep the water out of the generator room. That was a success as it meant we could keep things running. I don't think the maintenance staff that worked that day and night slept a wink; they were true heroes.

The medical aspects of that day were remarkable: triaging the hospital patients to determine who would be evacuated first if and when the time came; taking part in a helicopter transfer for two maternity patients who were in labour and seeing them off safely to fully equipped hospitals, which in the midst of the floods we most definitely were not; being flown back to High River Hospital by the military in a Griffin helicopter because that is where we were most useful (we had the opportunity to use their night-vision goggles to see the town under water, as a Hercules plane circled above us dropping flares to light the way back); and returning to the hospital, as some of the water receded, to assist nurses and medics in resuscitating a man in his seventies who was poorly responsive and hypothermic after being found in the freezing water. I remember pausing for a brief second before blurting out, "I'm a physician, can I help?" There are epic moments in life when you leap into the next phase of your journey and your training allows you to help someone in acute distress—this was one of mine.

High River is a town of resilient people. They have seen floods before, and they will see them again in the future. However, this flood was different. The speed at which the river rose, the speed at which the river flowed down the streets, shocked even veteran observers. No one had a chance to think twice, and if you did, you got caught in the current. We watched police boats drive up the streets only to flip against the current. We saw cars float down the streets rather than drive. We watched rescuers in front-end loaders and combines go window to window to evacuate people.

Finally, by 3 a.m. on Saturday, June 22, the High River Hospital evacuation was complete.

In the days and months to come, the town and its community members slowly began rebuilding their homes and places of work. The medical community of High River was severely affected. Multiple offices were destroyed and thankfully rebuilt, although it took longer than many of us expected. We worked together to support each other and to provide workspace so that patients could continue to be cared for. The hospital opened its doors to the local specialists so they could resume seeing patients as soon as was possible. Surgery and obstetrical services resumed within two and a half months. We increased mental health services because we knew the worst, emotionally, was yet to come.

● ● ●

Today, I am proud to say that I have spent a large portion of my early career working in High River. It is more than the rural medicine it allows me to practise that pulls me back. It is the people, this community that is working hard to rebuild what they had as they try to stand by each other, that keeps me coming back. However, it will never be the same. It still feels somewhat deserted at times, but those who have stayed behind continue to support each other and do their best for their families and community. Being part of this entire journey has changed me not only as a physician but also at the core of who I am as a person, which is for the better. It has made me stronger. High River strong.

**ALBERTA**

# Dr. Joseph Westgeest

*Joseph Westgeest is originally from New Westminster, British Columbia, and is currently a medical student at the University of Alberta. He is a co-founder of Seniors Know, a nonprofit seniors' services organization, and of the Edmonton chapter of Friends of Médecins Sans Frontières/Doctors Without Borders. Before entering medical school, Joseph worked extensively with seniors and special needs youth and adults. Outside of medicine, Joseph loves backcountry hiking and camping in both his home province of British Columbia, as well as throughout Alberta. He looks forward to gaining a new perspective on the mountains as he works towards his private pilot licence after graduation. Joseph lives in Edmonton, Alberta.*

## To Maury

"Watch out for Maury."

I had been at the local hospital for two weeks, but I hadn't met Maury. Nurses warned me of him, often with a wry smile. Even the cocksure senior resident changed the subject when I mentioned him. "He's a bit feisty," he said hurriedly, between charts. But I still hadn't met Maury.

I was a second-year medical student, and this small, northern, Alberta town was home for another three weeks while I completed my rural medicine elective. The goal was to gain some clinical experience while experiencing life in the countryside.

My time in the community so far had been lovely, punctuated by delightful riverside walks, suspiciously friendly townsfolk, and the uninterrupted beauty of my rural landscape. Each morning on my way to the hospital, the trees eased and bowed in the breeze, chattering noisily above the fallen leaves that carpeted my path with deep hues of amber, crimson, and brown. It was sublime.

The quiet, unassuming Ms. Dales was my first patient that day. "Anything I should know?" I asked my preceptor, Dr. Swanson.

"You tell me. Just do your usual and let me know if you find anything interesting. She's going to long-term care at the end of the week and I don't want any surprises once we get her there."

"My usual" consisted of interrogating hostage patients for the better part of an hour, quizzing them ungracefully before haltingly regurgitating my findings to an exasperated supervising doctor. It was a messy affair that I tried my best to conceal from anyone within earshot, especially staff. But I suspected Dr. Swanson was referring to completing a proper patient history and physical exam. I headed dutifully down the hall.

A housekeeper was exiting room 405. "Have you met Maury yet?" he asked. I hadn't. He smiled knowingly, connoting both pity and pleasure at my impending encounter. There was an apex predator on ward 3C, all right, and it wasn't the senior resident.

I knocked hesitantly on the door. Bedsheet-draped toes swayed along melodically to classical piano music as a tattered sunflower peered in from the window ledge. I entered the room.

Ms. Dales was a slight woman no more than forty years of age. Soft curled wisps of blond hair bestowed themselves on her shoulders. Her anonymous green gown belied the warmth that seemed to radiate from her every pore. Smiling, she looked up at me, paused, and breathed "welcome" with such conviction and warmth that I felt as if my kindly Polish grandmother herself had proclaimed it. I was immediately at ease.

I began my ritual. But I could soon tell that something wasn't quite right with Ms. Dales. Her arms curled up awkwardly towards her shoulders, and she seemed to have difficulty sitting still. Her fingers curled inwards, forming a fist. She spoke slowly and deliberately, meanwhile trying to catch the errant bits of drool that dribbled ungracefully from her mouth. I continued my history, but it was now more a question period than conversation. I tried to conceal my unease, but Ms. Dales could sense my growing distance. I had never before interviewed a patient with cognitive difficulties, and my inexperience showed. The conversation that followed only widened that divide.

"I just have a few more questions for you before we wrap up, Ms. Dales. As you know, Dr. Swanson will be transferring you to long-term care at the end of the week. I know that this isn't your preference, but Dr. Swanson informed me that there aren't any other options. In fact, you're lucky that a spot came up. As you know, beds are pretty tight, especially in rural areas like this." I looked up to see a tear pass down her cheek. Unsure how to react, I continued. "I just need to...."

"Perhaps we can continue tomorrow afternoon. Mornings aren't so good for me," she said, avoiding eye contact. I agreed.

I looked back as I left the room. No melodically swaying toes, and no more music. I moved on to my next patient, but my mind didn't follow.

I'm an optimist; I brought a stethoscope to my first autopsy. But my optimism couldn't overcome what we both knew: that long-term care was a terrible option for her. She would share a space with people twice her age. Ms. Dales was naturally sociable and would have no trouble making friends, but for what? Every few years, her relationships would end in heartache—old age is the great equalizer, and Ms. Dales was no equal. But there didn't seem to be a better option.

I returned the next day and entered Ms. Dales's room. Only this time, Maury was waiting.

His eyes seemed to glow in the darkness. His hair was shaggy and unkempt, and despite his diminutive frame, he was every bit as menacing as I expected. Breathing slowly and deliberately, he made no attempt to conceal his contempt for me. He shot me a knowing glance—perhaps he had learned of the botched history? But before I could explain my case, he lunged.

Immediately, I was transformed. I scanned the room frantically for IV poles, stools, furniture—anything I could jump on to save myself from the maniacal beast closing in on me.

"Maury! *Maury*!! Get *back* here!" Ms. Dales bellowed. As quickly as it began, the madness ceased. "I'm so sorry. He seems to do that to everybody," she said sweetly. He trotted back to the foot of her bed, circled, and lay down. He supervised me carefully.

"Nice dog," I stammered. As my trembling subsided, I worried that moisture quite different from that on my brow had already appeared on my pants. I didn't look.

"Well, perhaps we can finish that discussion we started yesterday, Ms. Dales." A low, rumbling growl was the prelude to the glistening, jagged teeth that followed. Maury's gums quivered. "Or maybe I can speak with Dr. Swanson about some alternatives to long-term care."

"That would be lovely," Ms. Dales said cheerfully. I promised to report back the following day. Maury seemed to nod sagely in agreement.

I thought about a lot that night, and my thoughts always seemed to come back to Maury. It was a shame, really, that more patients didn't have dogs—something to give patient advocacy some teeth. Perhaps all of medicine needs a little pet therapy.

# Dr. Andrew Lodge

*Andrew Lodge grew up on the Prairies before heading out on his own just after his seventeenth birthday for China, where he stayed for two years. Since then, he has spent time all over Canada and the world. He currently lives, works, and writes in the remote and predominantly Aboriginal community of Bella Coola, British Columbia, tucked away in the majestic Coast Mountains of the province's rugged west coast. In his capacity as a physician, he has taught and practised medicine in several different corners of the planet. Meanwhile, his writing has appeared in various publications both nationally and internationally. He has also co-directed a documentary about sex workers and the struggle against HIV/AIDS in rural India.*

## John Prine, Loneliness, and a Heart Attack

"I think he's having a heart attack."

The voice on the phone was Jeanette's, the nurse working the night shift. The urgency in her tone was palpable.

I rolled over in bed, the phone still at my ear. I had answered it in my sleep and was only waking up now.

"Mmmm," I replied. I sat up, trying to clear my head. "Could you give him some aspirin and get an ECG? I'll be right over."

I threw on a shirt and pants while pulling my boots on over my bare feet.

Outside the rain turned to sleet and obscured the mountains surrounding the remote First Nations town. Deep in the valley, we were the only people left in the world. The few visible streetlights were shrouded in a surreal haze.

I hurried over to the small hospital across the street from my house. The doors welcomed me and slid open as I walked into the dimly lit hall. I could see brightness emanating from the emergency room.

Jeanette met me at the entranceway and handed me the ECG; unmistakable ST segment elevation. She was right. He was having a heart attack, quite possibly a massive one.

He lay on the stretcher clutching his chest. He looked sweaty and gasped a bit but managed a "hey, Doc" when he saw me. As with everyone else in town, I was on a first-name basis with him. He was big and strong, an Aboriginal man known to be a good fisherman.

Jeanette was speaking.

"His vitals are normal, except for his respiratory rate." I already had a tourniquet on his left arm and slid an IV cannula in. She did the same on the other side.

I listened to the cursory story from him between his laboured breaths. It sounded just as it looked.

"Let's get ready to thrombolyze him," I said to her as she was hanging a bag of fluid for the IV. I tried to sound calm. This was the first thrombolysis I had faced since arriving in this remote community, the first one I had to do alone, hours upon hours from any sort of help should things go sideways.

I went through the contraindications and convinced myself there couldn't be another diagnosis. I checked the pulse and blood pressure in both arms. Jeanette called the lab and X-ray technicians, but they were both over thirty minutes away, maybe more with the bad weather.

We would go ahead without them.

I looked at the patient. "You'll be all right," I said and put a hand on his knee. I explained what was going on and what we had to do. He nodded.

"Do yer thing, Doc," he grunted. I could hear John Prine's guitar singing quietly overhead on the PA system. Jeanette must have had it playing before the patient arrived.

All set, I drew up the drug and stuck the needle into the port. I felt my own heart pounding as I pushed the medication into his veins. We watched the monitor and we watched him. The seconds ticked by interminably, but he slowly started to relax. Finally, after what seemed like hours—but was only a few minutes—he managed a wan smile.

"Pain's goin'," he said as he lay his head back.

• • •

It was quiet again and things had stabilized. Jeanette and I sat back in the swivel chairs behind the nursing station. The patient was parked, propped up on the stretcher in the hall beside us, just a short distance away, monitor beside him and IVs running slowly. He looked comfortable and smiled over at me when he saw me looking at him.

"I'll get that room ready across from here," Jeanette motioned to the room with a large window looking out to the nursing station—our intensive care unit, in a quaint sort of way. "That way I can watch him and the monitor tonight."

I nodded. We both fell silent. I took a sip from the cup of coffee the lab technician had made after she had finally arrived.

"But it's far, far from me...." Prine's voice drifted through the hall of the quiet little hospital.

"Hey, Doc, can you turn that up just a bit?" I looked over at our man on the stretcher, who was waiting patiently.

"Sure thing," I nodded. I pushed the chair across the nursing station to the desktop computer, which sat just beside his stretcher.

He lay back on the angled mattress. I glanced at him. Everything looked okay.

"Reminds me of my wife, ya know? She loved Johnny Prine." He was silent for a moment. "She died in this hospital years ago." He took a deep breath. "Thought I was joining her tonight. We weren't gettin' along so good back then. I got a few things I never had a chance to say to her." I looked over at him. Suddenly, there were tears streaming down his face. "Nice things, ya know?"

His eyes met mine and he took another deep breath.

"Things I shoulda said but didn't." I stepped over and squeezed his shoulder with my hand.

"Sometimes I get so lonely." His body shuddered and he leaned forward and pushed his head into my chest.

There was nothing else to do, no textbook section on this acute complication of myocardial infarction, so I just stood there and held him.

• • •

Things take time in a small hospital, tasks that one might take for granted elsewhere. I thought of the last heart attack I had managed, back in a larger town of eighty thousand people, with a small army of specialists and legions of nurses. I had written the orders and the drugs were given and my role was completed; my part in the whole rigmarole had taken maybe an hour, and I was gone.

I don't remember that patient's name.

It was a bit different in a one-horse town of two thousand, with the closest cardiac referral centre twelve hours away on a ridiculously terrifying mountain road.

Together, Jeanette and I put a new sheet on the bed. I helped her wheel the patient and then his monitor into the room. We brought the crash cart over just as a safety measure.

Just as we were finishing this up, the entrance doors to the hospital slid open. I braced myself for another patient at this late hour. It didn't take much to overload our capacity.

But it was the man's son, who had somehow heard the news and had come in to check on his father. I knew they had been estranged for years and wondered what was up. Nevertheless, I pointed him to his father's room and he walked on in.

By the time the remainder of the cardiac cocktail of pills had been given, his lines checked, the charting all finished, and orders clarified, it was almost morning. I looked through the ICU window one last time. The man was asleep in his bed. He had been for some time. In the chair beside him, his son had fallen asleep as well. I could see they were holding hands as they slept. The monitor did its blinking thing.

I left the hospital but skipped the going-back-to-bed step and instead walked down the road to the local diner—the only game in town—for another coffee.

The air was crisp and cool, the ground was wet, but it had stopped sleeting.

John Prine's voice played in my head. Not surprising. It had played on a loop all night. Our man and his son had sung along softly together until, one by one, they had fallen asleep.

Medicine for the soul, or at least for his.

# Dr. Julia Low Ah Kee

*Julia Low Ah Kee was born and raised a suburban British Columbia girl and never thought that she would end up a BC, BC, girl—that is, a girl who lives in Bella Coola, British Columbia. After choosing the University of British Columbia's Rural Residency Family Medicine training program and a string of fortuitous events, she found her husband in Bella Coola, where she has learned to harvest meat (including moose, deer, salmon, halibut, crab, and prawns), grow fruit and vegetables, appreciate drinking fresh glacier water, and fill the woodshed to keep warm in the winter. She loves the good clean living, where her children can still play outside and the biggest threat is the wildlife. She is happiest hearing about her children's day at the dinner table, which can include stories of swimming in the pond and catching newts before going for a horseback ride and gathering chicken eggs. She can't think of a better life.*

## Goldibear and the Four Anglers

"*Run!!!*" Lawrence yelled, as the grizzly started bounding up the hillside towards us. A minute earlier, I had spotted the bear as I crested over the knoll, only to see my husband trudging down the second switchback, head down, towards our fishing hole, not noticing the giant, golden-brown head turn slowly in our general direction. Behind her, I saw a solitary black ball of fur crossing a log towards her. Uh-oh, I thought, only one cub; that's not good news…she will be extra protective.

"Lawrence…there's…a…bear." I tried to whisper softly but forcefully so he would hear me, but not so loud as to alert the grizzly to our presence if she had not yet seen us. My heart was pounding because we had no protection. Just bear spray, which he often joked would be like seasoning ourselves with fresh pepper before serving ourselves to the grizzly.

"Go…back…up…back up," Lawrence mouthed exaggeratedly, as he waved his brother-in-law Vern, Too Tall Phil, and I back up over the knoll, hoping to sneak away without having the bear notice us. We were too late; she had seen us sometime between when I saw her look up and us turning to sneak away. Unhappy bear eyes noted that we had the nerve to encroach upon her space, especially with her lone cub, at *her* fishing hole. Too Tall Phil bolted. After being bent over his knees every few steps on the hike in, he had gotten an adrenaline boost and taken off into the woods with three-metre strides. Of all of us, he could have just stood still and the bear would have mistaken him for a tree, so skinny and tall he was.

So there we were, frantically running up the hill, being charged by an angry grizzly sow. Completely helpless, with no protection except bear spray, whose futility an old-timer imparted to me when he explained, "Might as well fart at 'em."

I turned to look back at Lawrence as I was running and caught a vision that has since been the premise of a few bad dreams. His eyes were as wide as saucers—he looked like he had severe Graves' disease—and the panic in his face as he scrambled up the hill towards me showed me he knew what could soon hit him. The grizzly bounded swiftly up the hill, ears back in a full charge, with a speed I could not have imagined possible for such a massive beast.

"Give me the bear spray!" Lawrence shouted. I fumbled at my waist belt and shoved the virgin can into his hands. He turned towards the bear, stood his ground, and started roaring loudly at her, getting ready to spray her with perfume and say his final Hail Mary. Vern and I stopped a ways behind him and followed his lead, hollering at her and grabbing rocks and clacking them together like barbarians.

The sow stopped less than three metres short of contact, either bewildered or impressed by our valiant display of courage. She reared up on her back legs, threw up some dirt in a hissy fit, turned a sharp ninety degrees away, and thrashed into the woods, her little black cub on her heels.

Nobody talked as we stood there, panting heavily, partly from the uphill sprint but mostly from the adrenaline rush of almost being eaten by a bear and not having any control over it. Helpless; I have never felt so powerless in my life. The prevailing thought going through my mind in that frantic moment was, "Shit, this is it. I hope it doesn't hurt." Eloquent, but you don't have much time to choose your words when you're faced with death so starkly.

I thought about my brush with death over the next while as we fished a different hole. My thoughts must not have been so different from those of my two palliative patients in town, whose life stories could not have been more distinct. Mrs. Bruce was a Caucasian spinster—she literally spun wool—in her late eighties, the wife of an old pioneer rancher whose hard-working family had earned themselves a road named after them on the Chilcotin Plateau. She was a devoted wife, riding the community bus daily to the hospital to visit her ailing husband in long-term care. That is, until her struggle with anemia and chronic cough ended up being metastatic lung cancer that had spread to her liver and bones. Now it was her turn to have her family visit her in her home, where she lived independently and wanted to stay until the end. But even at the last home visit, she was still not ready to talk about death but was content exchanging pleasantries instead. She was just happy that she was comfortable.

Ms. Talon was a First Nations lady in her early fifties who would make anyone believe that the creator (whoever you believe the creator to be) was having a bad day when they devised her life story. In early life, she was sickened with rheumatic heart disease that proceeded to complicate her life with atrial fibrillation in her forties. She suffered a gigantic, right-sided stroke that underwent hemorrhagic transformation, requiring craniotomies and ultimately the removal of a large part of her right skullcap. In addition to the dense left hemiparesis, she suffered from chronic infections from her numerous cranioplasties. On top of all that, while in hospital for another repair, one of her care providers decided to investigate her oligomenorrhea only to discover inoperable cervical cancer. With neurosurgery, plastic surgery, gynecological oncology, oncology, psychiatry, and physiatry all signing off, where else was there to go but back home to Bella Coola, where she had not lived for years but wished to return to for her final days. She refused to acknowledge them as her final days, but those around her could not help but see it. They cared for her lovingly with traditional Aboriginal medicine, rubbing a concoction of bear grease (rendered grizzly bear fat), comfrey, pine, birch, and numerous other ingredients all over her body to ease the contractures of her left limbs, as well as on her open scalp wounds, without batting an eye. But no amount of drum dancing in her room could change her final outcome.

Though our stories could not be more dissimilar, we did have one thing in common. When I looked into their eyes, I knew what they were thinking. It was the same thought I had when I was running for my life. "Shit, this is it. I hope it doesn't hurt." However, the difference was that in their lives, I was not nearly as powerless as I was with regards to my own brush with death.

I could try to make it not hurt for them. Though I did not have the ability to change their ultimate outcome, I was able to ease their journey's end. I learned that it was a noble task not only to relieve pain but also to allay the fear of pain.

**BRITISH COLUMBIA**

# Dr. Warren Bell

*Born and raised in Vancouver, British Columbia, and having gradu-*
*ated and completed his residency at McGill University, Warren Bell*
*has been a family physician for over thirty-eight years. For over three*
*decades he has been actively involved in issues of social development,*
*including the environment, the peace and antinuclear movement, and*
*global health and development with an emphasis on the role of multi-*
*national drug companies. Many of these topics were addressed in a*
*weekly newspaper column he wrote entitled Global Health. He is a*
*past president of Physicians for Global Survival and the Association*
*of Complementary and Integrative Physicians of BC. He was the*
*founding president of the Canadian Association of Physicians for the*
*Environment and was for five years president of the medical staff of the*
*Shuswap Lake General Hospital. Currently, he resides in a small town*
*in south-central British Columbia, running an active practice that*
*integrates conventional and alternative or complementary remedies.*

## Instant Immersion

My startling introduction to practicing small-town medicine occurred in Salmon Arm, British Columbia, on July 1,
1979—nearly thirty-five years ago.

Prior to moving to this community, I lived in Vancouver and Montreal—hardly what you would call rural settings. My entire medical experience had been with big-city medicine, except for one notable two-week stint in the village of Ormstown, Quebec, during my family medicine training. There, I learned a lot about small-town pragmatism, such as office vasectomies performed by the local surgeon on Fridays so patients could return to work on Mondays! I knew I wanted to work in a rural setting, where I felt I could be a "real" doctor using "real" skills.

We moved back to British Columbia after I had worked three years in the emergency room of the Queen Elizabeth Hospital in Montreal. My wife and I wanted to be back in Lotusland, where we had both been born and where our aging parents needed more attention.

I will admit we found the winter weather and scenery a lot more attractive as well.

And…there was a position advertised in a clinic in Salmon Arm.

Initially, I travelled alone across the country by plane to begin work. My wife stayed behind in Montreal to organize the sale of our home—selling into a market monumentally depressed by the recent election of René Lévesque and the Parti Québécois. Needless to say, it was a slow process to sell our home.

Arriving in Salmon Arm in a rented car, having driven from the airport in Kelowna, I was greeted by a senior member of the clinic I was joining. He warmly welcomed me and took me to his home and introduced me to his wife and to his brother-in-law visiting from Edmonton.

That's where I made my first mistake.

My new colleague was, shall we say, socially conservative, but his brother-in-law was…well, let me just say his neck was a pretty shade of crimson. Anxious and nervous about being in a new situation, and fresh from life in a large urban centre, I burbled on, heedlessly airing my "liberal" points of view.

I was met with increasingly stony silence from the brother-in-law.

Eventually receiving the message, I clammed up. Supper featured a sustained and intermittent discussion of local meteorological matters.

After dinner, the plates were as cold as the conversation. I was then taken to the home of another physician, the founder of the clinic I was joining. He was leaving town for holidays with his family and had generously given me the run of his home while he was away.

As I was being dropped off, my supper host informed me I would be on call—including emergency coverage—for the three days spanning the Canada Day holiday weekend. All of my new colleagues, all five, would be leaving town.

I was it.

I gulped internally and went to bed for an uneasy, restless night.

The next three days and nights were a blur. I was called frequently to the emergency room, fortunately for problems that were within my comfort zone. I saw a bevy of my new partners' in-patients, and tried desperately to remember where everything was in the Shuswap Lake General Hospital, my new professional home. All weekend long, I learned and then forgot and then relearned the names of key staff.

Then I was called to attend a delivery.

A word of explanation: my training in obstetrics at McGill had been abysmally light. The six-week rotation had involved me observing a dozen births, each involving the lithotomy position and leg straps, an intravenous, an episiotomy, and forceps without much in the way of analgesia and anesthesia. I don't recall even putting on a pair of gloves.

Certainly, I was terrified of having to use forceps after listening to the cries of birthing women on whom they were being employed. I felt I had hardly any idea of how to handle complications—which, thanks to the somewhat pathology-focused atmosphere in the case room of a large teaching hospital, I was sure would be the secret centrepiece of most births.

Another of my new associates had cheerily told me, as he was heading out the door and out of town—*way* out of town—"Don't worry, most babies just deliver themselves. And if you need any help, there is always lots of backup."

Except that all the backup had just joyously disappeared on vacation.

As it turned out, the baby did deliver herself. I watched, trembling and filled with dire fantasies, smiling and thinking of old reruns of *Marcus Welby, M.D.*, doing my best to project an image of casual and concerned competency. As the birth progressed smoothly and uneventfully, it gradually became clear that I was relatively and reassuringly redundant. The nurses knew all the routines, all the forms and documents, and where everything was in the case room. I just had to smile sweetly and avoid dropping the baby on the floor, as well as listen carefully to the diplomatic suggestions from the nurses—things like, "Well, I guess it's time to cut the cord, isn't it?"

As in many previous moments during my residency—and since—I offered private thanks to the Great Goddess of Nursing for saving my bacon. After the birth was completed, I lavished more overt thanks on the nurses involved.

Terror is a wonderful thing.

I rushed off and began reviewing everything I could about childbirth.

Over the next twenty-five years, delivering a few hundred babies, I learned a great deal and eventually became known as the local "quasi-midwife." I can even say I read *Spiritual Midwifery* by Ina May Gaskin—not because of the volume of births I attended, but because of the care and attention I put into keeping up-to-date and deliberately advancing beyond the antediluvian precepts that had filled my head when I arrived in the rural setting.

After that first weekend, everything seemed pretty tame. I went to work in the clinic, saw in-patients at the hospital, did emergency shifts, assisted at major surgeries, made an occasional home visit—and delivered babies with increasing confidence.

My wife sold our home in Montreal and joined me in Salmon Arm in first a rented house, and then in the very conventional home we bought at the absolute peak of the real estate market in British Columbia for almost exactly the same price that we sold our three-storey home with hardwood floors, solid oak woodwork, a marble fireplace, and stained-glass ornaments in Montreal.

I quickly decided against a secondary career in real estate.

Over the next few months, it became clear there were tensions in the clinic. One physician had few formal appointments, lots of drop-ins and add-ons, and was terrible at keeping up on his charts, which piled up in stacks in his office and examining rooms. His two colleagues were organized, kept strict schedules, had very few drop-ins, and moved patients briskly in and out of their offices.

I presented a whole other problem. I was at the time finishing a paper on the *CPS—The Compendium of Pharmaceuticals and Specialties*—still the only detailed research paper in the medical literature on the subject. In the course of my research, I had learned a great deal about the pharmaceutical industry and was highly skeptical of its intentions and wary of its influence.

Yet in the clinic, practically every storage cupboard was overflowing with free pharmaceutical samples. Now widely accepted as marketing loss leaders, back then they were considered an essential component of office practice.

Inevitably, comments would pass about the role of the drug industry, or even about the role of the medical profession itself.

I was clearly trouble.

The denouement of these tensions, for me, came in the form of a confrontation no more than six or seven months after I had arrived in town.

The head of the clinic asked me to follow one of his terminally ill patients at home on the weekend. I had worked in palliative care for two years at the Royal Victoria Hospital in Montreal and was confident of my skills.

But when I saw this patient, I found out my colleague had told him that since he was eating little, we would start a D5W (5 per cent dextrose in water) intravenous for him at home. From two years in palliative care, I knew this was not going to be helpful, but I nevertheless made several attempts to start an IV. The patient's veins were fragile, and every attempt resulted in a blowout. So I talked to him and his family about sips of fluids, keeping his mouth moist with swabs, and all the other tricks I had learned over the previous two years.

The patient was quite happy with this arrangement. But when the clinic head returned to town, he was furious. And so a few weeks later, he came around to our home and informed my wife and I that I would have to leave the clinic.

I was devastated. I had never worked in a small town before, and now, barely eight months after arriving, I was being cut loose. I had no idea what to do but imagined leaving town with my tail between my legs.

Then an angel arrived.

The only surgeon in town, a large-framed, bluff gent who also, fortuitously, happened to be McGill-trained, invited us over for supper and told us bluntly that the obvious solution was to open my own office.

He then went on to point out that the clinic founder—the one who had fired me—had done precisely the same thing when he arrived in town, after being rebuffed by the other clinic already in town. In fact, he had established his first office in a downtown hotel room!

Encouraged by this, and by a few other contacts in the community outside the medical profession, we decided to stay and make this place home. I rented space, and my wife and I renovated it over several exhausting weeks. We opened up, and to my astonishment and delight, almost all the patients I had seen in the clinic—even patients I had seen once and only for a minor problem—sought us out and came to the new office. I was overwhelmed with gratitude and a renewed sense of confidence.

I've now worked in this solo practice for nearly thirty-five years, sharing coverage with other physicians in the community. My wife was a much-appreciated office manager until two years ago. The advantages of a working in one's own office are not often touted these days: the intellectual freedom, the engagement that comes from having patients coming specifically to see you, and the detailed understanding of their lives built up over years.

The fractured relationships with my former colleagues have warmed and rebalanced over the years. Practitioners have come and gone, facilities have been rebuilt and changed hands, and daily practices have steadily evolved. And the population of our town has doubled.

It's been a ride, but I have absolutely no regrets. Moving to a small town to practise was the best decision I made in my professional career.

# Dr. Robert James Henderson

*Robert Henderson was born in London, Ontario, and grew up nearby in the rural village of Lambeth. He attended school locally, received a degree in biology, and was accepted into medicine at the University of Western Ontario. He met and married Wendy in 1967 and they had three children, who now live with their families in British Columbia. He interned in Victoria and then moved to Vernon, where from 1973 to 2000 he maintained a full-time family practice, including obstetrics and ER coverage. That experience proved invaluable when, switching paths in 2000, he moved to rural locums on Gabriola Island. Currently, he is pushing for greater recognition of the importance of rural locums in the survival of rural medicine as we know it. In an attempt to promote a spreading of knowledge and better communication, he helped to create the first annual Rural Locum Conference, which was held in February 2015 in Nanaimo, BC.*

## Where the Buck Stops

Sixteen years ago, I was burnt out.

I had long realized that, at least for me, better medicine meant more time with each patient. The terrible irony of that reduced patient volume meant more pressure from more people who wanted good, caring medicine, which meant more stress and almost the lowest gross income in my community in the Okanagan Valley. I loved medicine, but it was driving me crazy.

I joined the GP rural locum program of British Columbia, found someone to take over my practice, and moved to Gabriola Island.

Through the program, I was fortunate enough to come to do locums on that beautiful island, but also on Hornby Island. I had many acquaintances who travelled to Hornby each summer to vacation, and I had wondered what it would be like to practise medicine on a small island. Suddenly, I had the opportunity to do lots of locums, because the blind determination of the regional health managers at that time to have a solo doctor work 24/7/365 meant that the community had lost its long-time family doctor. Also, working alone in those circumstances scares the hell out of most urban doctors, and no permanent solution was about to occur, so locum doctors flowed through Hornby Island like water over a fall, with nary a chance to get to know the community.

When no locum physician could be found, a kind and smart rural-trained nurse, who lives on the island, filled in brilliantly. The islanders had no idea how fortunate they were, and through her, I was allowed to discover how committed, caring, rural nurses can have as much, or more, influence on the well-being of the citizens. Daily in rural communities, they skilfully go about saving lives. Our nurse did not only that, but did palliative care, wound management, and guided patient rehabilitation. When I eventually realized that I had found my second home, I felt like I was practising the best kind of medicine that I could possibly imagine, making "rounds" by car to visit the sick, wounded, and dying by myself, or often with our nurse.

A wonderful aspect about this was that a contract had been created with the health authority. I convinced them to split the service contract, built a house, and took on a 0.5 full-time equivalent position. People used to say I was only working half-time. That "halftime" was 24/7 for 182 days of the year. When working, I always had a pager, never left the island, and, in fact, was never more than about fifteen minutes from the clinic, even when running or mountain biking the trails. The official contract was for 37.5 hours weekly. That did not include nights, holidays, and weekends. There was no after-hours funding, and none for looking after nonclinic patients. The island population grew from one thousand through the winter to six thousand, at least at peak times in August. When asked how patients would be looked after if I chose to only work 37.5 hours a week, the answer was by whatever means possible.

I was able to practise medicine at my pace, with little office overhead, and for people who often gave you a hug before they sat down to tell you their troubles. The people would either phone the pager directly or would call 911, and ambulance dispatch would page the doctor, a situation that must be very rare in British Columbia, but it worked well, and I would often be on-scene before the first responders, which made sense as, beyond rescue and basic life support, they had little training.

The residents were mostly wonderful, bright, interesting people, often a bit quirky, but with minds full of art and designs. Everybody walked, almost no one was obese, there was absolutely no drug seeking. One time, I arranged to have a nurse specializing in diabetes come over, and it was a big stretch even in this community with a number of older patients to find twenty-five diabetics.

Yes, I could be called out at any time. Yes, I had to look at my watch when an urgent call happened in order to think about when the next ferry would be leaving and whether I would need to delay its departure. Yes, if I failed, the patient might die, but if I was not there, death could be a likely outcome.

Sending a patient off-island after the ferries shut down for the night was a big cost, whether the ferries needed to be called out or a helicopter was needed. Initially, this was something I thought about, but the reality was that no matter the $3,000–$4,000 cost, there was no alternative. The ferry crew never grumbled about being called out. These patients were friends and neighbours, or complete strangers from Washington state. Everyone was treated equally. The acute hemorrhage from an ulcer or a missed abortion, the anaphylaxis, the severe asthmatic—they were all treated and stabilized as well as possible before transport. By helicopter or ferry, it was at least ninety minutes before another doctor was going to lay hands on my patient.

I carried IV fluids, needles, and lines, as did the first responder vehicle. Since we had no paramedics on our island, my kit also included ambu bags, oxygen, and a large tackle box full of drugs. For many years we had no defibrillator. We had a big, old ECG machine at the office.

The reality was that the island and the people were amazing, but the clinic was a disaster! When I arrived, the cramped, old, double-wide trailer that housed the clinic had old carpet everywhere. There were two 60-watt light bulbs in the ER, which was about 2.5 x 2.5 metres in size, with so little room that you had to arrange the emergency table carefully so that you had access to the head or the feet, but not both at once. The patients were brought in through a side door via some very slippery steps and had to be turned sideways to get around a bookshelf that stood opposite to the door and only about a metre away. At night, everyone had to bring in a flashlight in case wounds needed to be examined or some suturing needed to be done.

Fairly shortly on, a midday storm knocked the power out. I asked what was to be done about seeing patients and was told that there was no emergency lighting and that the clinic simply shut down. These tales tell you why it was often easier to see an emergency on-site rather than in the clinic.

The examining table in the clinic was the old operating table from the emergency room. That was where every form of examination, including pelvic exams and Pap smears, was done. There was no means of putting the end of the table down to properly insert a speculum, so it had to be used upside down. I had done a lot of well-woman medicine and did not tolerate that situation for long. I ended up bringing down a used exam table from my old community, and it made life much easier for my patients and me. The lighting quickly got ripped out and much better lighting was installed. The bookshelf was also ripped out and shingles were nailed to the stairs. Through the regional district and the wonderful health care society, a generator was installed and we had lighting and heat no matter what happened. A few years later, that same society, through funds raised entirely on the island and with volunteer labour, built a wonderful new clinic for the community.

When not in the office, I was often out biking, running, or hiking the wonderful trails. I joined the art group and had occasional art shows, which was great fun.

The buck stops in a hurry in rural medicine. With a nurse, first responders, or even a medical student around, a lot can be done in a hurry—lives can be saved or serious illness cured.

The life of a rural doctor is an adventure. It is unlike urban medicine in most ways, and that is why it is such a wonderful experience. The challenges that come with that can be large at times, but the satisfaction of work well done is the best reward—I expect that the same is true across Canada.

# About the Editor

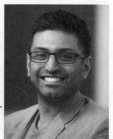

Photo: Diphile Iradukunda

Dr. Paul Dhillon practises full-scope rural medicine in Saskatchewan and is a Reservist Medical Officer in 16 Field Ambulance, Canadian Armed Forces. While completing his medical studies in Ireland, he self-published two books about a fictional Irish medical intern, and an excerpt from his first novel was the recipient of the Aindreas McEntee Irish Medical Writing Prize. Most recently he completed an overseas stint with Save the Children UK in the Kerry Town Ebola Treatment Centre and was the Senior Medical Authority for Exercise Arctic Ram in the Canadian High Arctic. He lives out of his Land Rover while traveling around the country and world with his wife, Sarah.